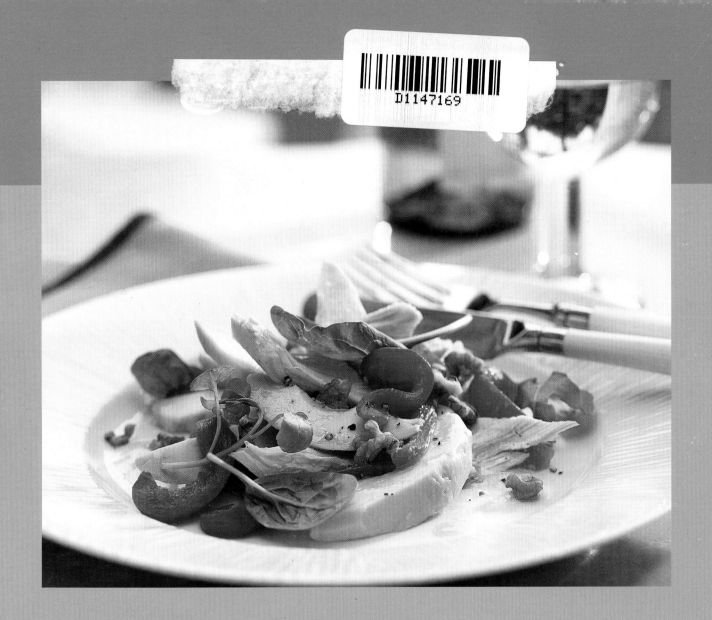

GREAT **HEALTHY** FOOD

DIABETES

AZMINA GOVINDJI

CARROLL & BROWN PUBLISHERS LIMITED

First published in 2001 in the United
Kingdom by:

Carroll & Brown Publishers Limited
20 Lonsdale Road
Queen's Park
London NW6 6RD

Editor Yvonne Deutch
Designer Justin Ford
Photographers David Murray
& Jules Selmes
Food Stylists Clare Lewis, Lizzie Harris
& Annie Nichols

Copyright © 2001
Carroll & Brown Limited

A CIP catalogue record for this book is
available from the British Library.

ISBN 1-903258-17-0

Reproduced by Colourscan, Singapore
Printed and bound in Great Britain by
The Bath Press
First edition

The moral right of Azmina Govindji to be
identified as the author of this work has
been asserted in accordance with the
Copyright, Designs and Patents Act of
1988.

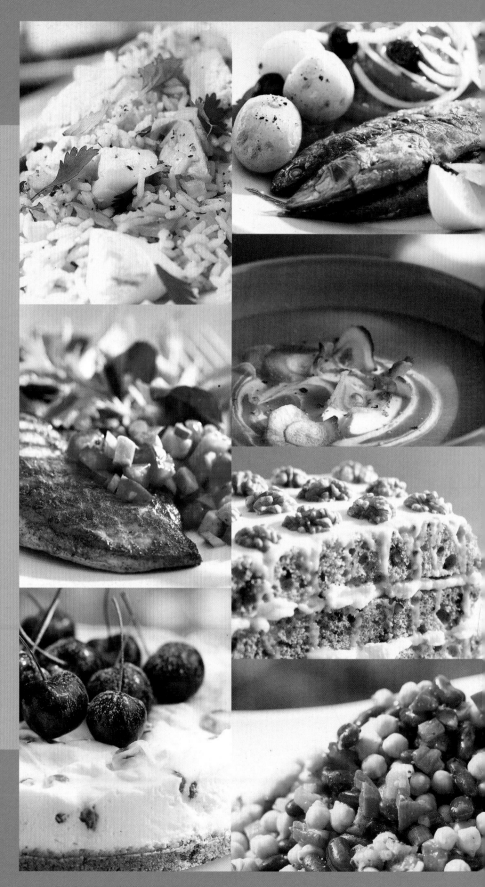

Contents

Introduction

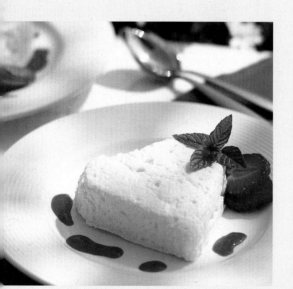

Eating is one of the great pleasures of life and there's no reason to miss out if you have diabetes. You can still enjoy an array of appetising and mouth-watering flavours and aromas, whilst making healthy choices for you and your family. This book will show you what you can eat, not give you a list of those foods you should avoid. The recipes are delicious and varied – you'll come across delights such as Monkfish Kebabs with Lemon and Thyme, and Turkey with Red Onion and Watercress Salad, along with traditional favourites like Stuffed Peppers and Mince Pies. You also can treat yourself with the Chocolate and Almond Custard Tart or the Banana Ice Cream with Chocolate and Hazelnut Topping.

WHAT THIS BOOK OFFERS

Each recipe featured in the book has been carefully tested using the latest guidelines for a diabetic diet – all of the meals and snacks combine a range of appropriate ingredients which help you to maintain steady glucose levels. Healthy eating, particularly for people with diabetes, is all about balance. It's also about being able to choose a variety of foods you enjoy and making them part of a healthy lifestyle that fits in with your current food preferences and eating habits – you don't need to completely change your diet.

Many of the recipes are based on the tempting tastes of the Mediterranean. Foods such as oily fish, garlic, olive oil, fruit and vegetables all play a part in the healthy Mediterranean diet, which research studies have found to have significant health benefits for diabetes. The recipes in this book have been specifically created so that you get the best out of these ingredients.

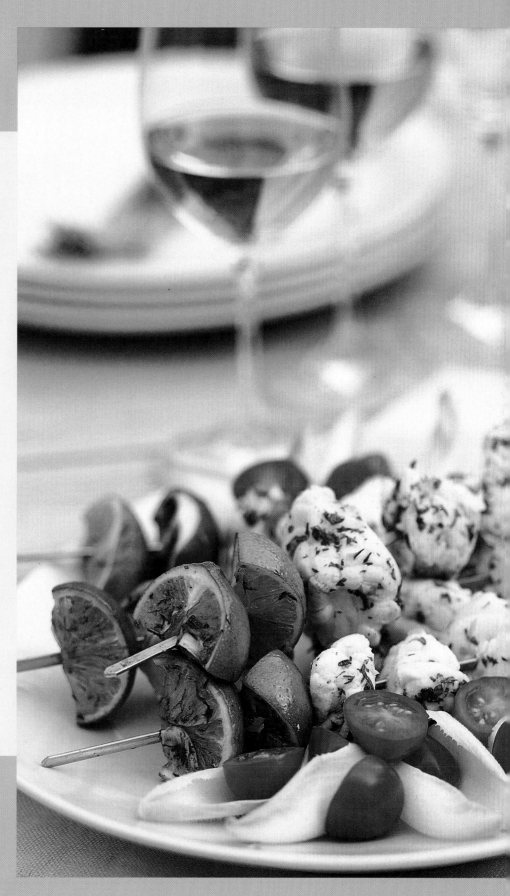

Some of the dishes featured in this book may, at first, appear to be absolute 'no-go areas' for people with diabetes. But let's dispel the myth that people with diabetes need a special diet. All foods can be incorporated into a healthy way of eating – it's getting the combinations right that's important. Rich chocolate desserts and main meals cooked in butter may sound totally out of the question, but remember that the recipes in this book have been created in line with healthy eating principles and generally use low-fat, low-calorie ingredients, such as reduced-fat spreads, fromage frais, light evaporated milk, and so on.

Each chapter in this book contains recipes for meals that will be enjoyed by family and friends, whether or not they have diabetes. You'll also notice some magnificent ideas for entertaining, so you can be sure that you're looking after your diet even when you're having fun with friends. Throughout, I've given recipe variations so you can enjoy different, yet equally delicious, creations.

WHAT IS DIABETES?

When you have diabetes, the amount of glucose in your blood is too high. Insulin, the hormone which helps glucose enter the cells where it is used as fuel by the body, is not produced in sufficient quantities by a person with diabetes. If there is not enough insulin, or if the insulin you have is not working well, then glucose can build up in your blood. This causes the symptoms of diabetes which are thirst, a dry mouth, passing large amounts of urine, loss of weight, tiredness, genital itchiness and blurred vision.

There are two kinds of diabetes: **Non insulin dependent diabetes** is the most common type. Here, the body can still make some insulin, but not enough for its needs. Non insulin dependent diabetes can be treated by a healthy diet alone, or by a combination of diet and tablets, or by diet and insulin injections. **Insulin dependent diabetes** occurs when the body is unable to produce its own insulin. It is treated with insulin injections, combined with a healthy diet.

The main aim of treatment is to avoid 'highs' and 'lows' in the body's blood glucose level. Together with a healthy lifestyle, this treatment will help to improve your well-being and protect against long-term damage to your eyes, kidneys, nerves and heart. There is no cure for diabetes, but with the appropriate treatment, you can enjoy a full, healthy and active life.

NUTRITIONAL GUIDELINES

Eat regular meals – this will help your blood glucose remain steady throughout the day, minimising potentially harmful highs and lows.

Try to get to a healthy weight and stay there – being overweight can put a strain on your body organs, especially the heart.

Select foods with a low glycaemic index – the latest research highlights the theory of Glycaemic Index (GI), which ranks foods according to how they affect blood glucose levels. The faster a food is broken down during digestion, the quicker blood glucose levels will rise. Foods that cause a rapid rise in blood glucose will have a high GI, so choose more foods with low GI's regularly. Foods which are high in soluble fibre, such as rye, granary and soft-grain white bread, peas, sweetcorn, beans, lentils, citrus fruits and oats have a low GI.

Make starchy foods (such as bread, potatoes, pasta, cereals and rice) the main part of your meal – starchy carbohydrates will help to fill you up, and tend to be lower in calories than fatty foods.

Cut down on fried and fatty foods such as butter, full-fat cheese, fatty meats, crisps and pastries – fats are an essential component of the diet, but too many saturated fats, found in meat and dairy products, can lead to a build up of fatty streaks in the arteries which can reduce blood flow to the heart.

Eat five portions of fruit and vegetables a day – fruit and vegetables contain vital anti-oxidant vitamins (A, C and E). Anti-oxidents protect against chemicals called free radicals, which, though formed naturally by the body, can cause damage and increase your risks of heart problems.

Swap high sugar foods (e.g. tinned fruit in syrup; sugar) for low sugar foods (e.g. tinned fruit in natural juice; artificial sweeteners) – high sugar foods cause glucose levels to rise quickly, so it is important to keep an eye on your sugar intake. It is, however, a misconception that people with diabetes should avoid sugar altogether. High sugar foods and drinks, consumed on an empty stomach, rapidly increase blood glucose. However, if sugar is eaten with other foods, especially at the end of a high fibre meal, the blood glucose rises more slowly, as this decreases the time it takes for the sugar to enter the bloodstream.

Eat more fish and have oily fish once a week – scientific studies suggest that oily fish may be protective against heart problems. Omega-3 oils, found in oily fish, have been shown to lower blood fats like cholesterol.

Choose foods which are low in salt – eating too much salt has been associated with high blood pressure and strokes. Most of the salt you eat comes from manufactured foods, such as bacon, canned fish and salted snack foods. Choose home-prepared foods where you have control over the amount of salt added.

THE IMPORTANCE OF DIET

What you eat is the most important part of any treatment for diabetes. Whether you need to take medication or not, the foods you choose and how often you eat have a significant effect on your blood glucose levels – watching your diet allows you to control the level of sugar in your blood. A low saturated fat diet is particularly beneficial for people with diabetes, who have an increased risk of developing heart disease. Remember that insulin or tablets are not a substitute for a healthy diet.

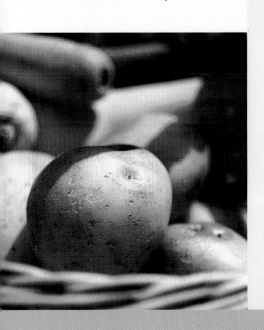

Chapter 1 helps you start the day with inspiring choices for breakfast, featuring recipes containing high fibre ingredients such as oats and fruit, as well as more unusual fish and egg dishes. Breakfast is an important meal of the day, especially as early-morning blood glucose levels may need stabalizing at this time.

In Chapter 2, you'll find a collection of light meals and snacks, including sandwiches, salads, jacket potatoes and pizza. It is often recommended that people with diabetes eat lighter meals regularly and often, so these recipes are ideal choices for food that can be eaten throughout the day. This chapter also introduces you to different breads, for example ciabatta and pitta, as well as giving away tricks of the trade, such as a lower-fat way of making popcorn.

Chapter 3 paves the way for the main meals to follow, featuring a varied selection of starters and warming soups, perfect for entertaining. These recipes have been created to release glucose into the blood stream gradually, to avoid blood glucose levels rising too quickly at the beginning of the meal.

You can afford to be adventurous with the meat, fish, poultry and vegetarian main courses in Chapter 4, as you'll be given step by step instructions on all the recipes, which include risottos, stir-fries and even home-made wraps. Cooking methods such as griddling, baking, pan-frying, grilling and boiling all go a long way to ensure that you keep the fat low, while preserving all the natural flavours and goodness of the carefully selected ingredients. This chapter also contains useful tips on starchy foods, such as polenta and couscous, allowing you to increase your repertoire for filling and tasty meals.

Chapter 5 presents you with ideas for many colourful vegetable dishes, along with many other accompaniments, which include beans, pulses and traditional Mediterranean favourites. Vegetables are a crucial part of a healthy diabetic

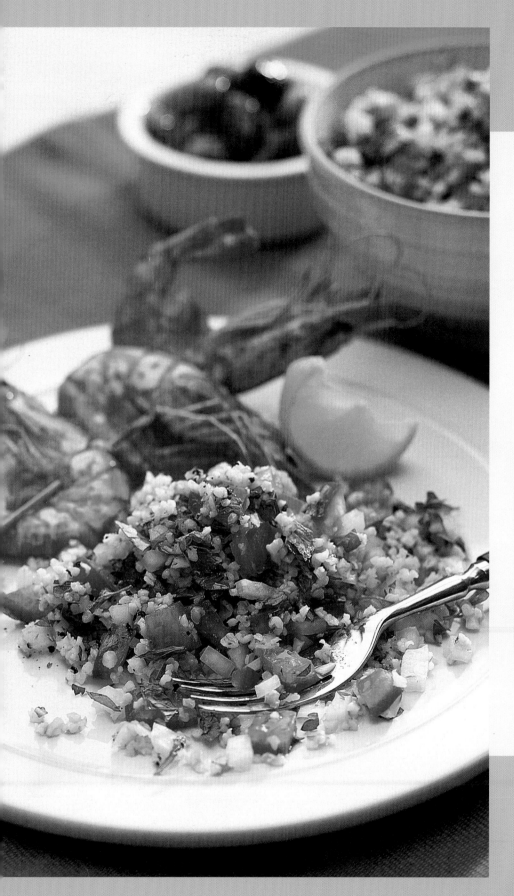

way of eating, as they provide essential vitamins and minerals and are high in fibre, which fills you up, helping to prevent weight gain – this is an important consideration for many people with diabetes.

Chapter 6 demonstrates that people with diabetes can enjoy a wide variety of delicious desserts, while maintaining a healthy diet. The hot, cold and iced desserts are oozing with ingredients like fresh raspberries, almonds, chocolate, lime, cinnamon, ginger and much more.

The cakes and breads in Chapter 7 will inspire you with quick and easy ways to conjure up your own treats for a special occasion or afternoon snack. This chapter includes recipes for granary bread, fruit scones, flapjacks, as well as a range of cakes and crunchy tea-time treats.

The recipes in this book demonstrate that a diabetic diet need not be limited or restrictive. Food in diabetes is all about the enjoyment of delicious ingredients and an appreciation of healthy eating. With quality Mediterranean ingredients combined in inventive, creative recipes that use healthy cooking methods, this book is your chance to have your cake and eat it, whether you have diabetes or not!

NOTES TO THE COOK

Most of the ingredients in this book will be available from your local supermarket or grocery store. To help you watch your fat intake, I've suggested using ingredients such as spray oil, fromage frais and low or reduced-fat spreads. Low-fat speads (which contain around 40 per cent fat) can contain too much water to be effective in some recipes, and so reduced-fat (70 per cent fat) spreads are used instead. It is, therefore, important to note which type of fat is listed in the ingredients. Where a recipe calls for salt, use the minimum possible and for pepper, choose freshly ground black pepper.

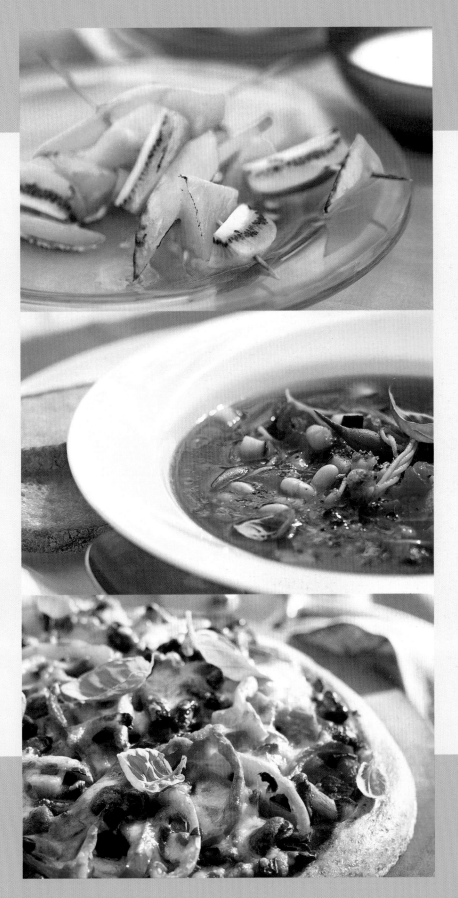

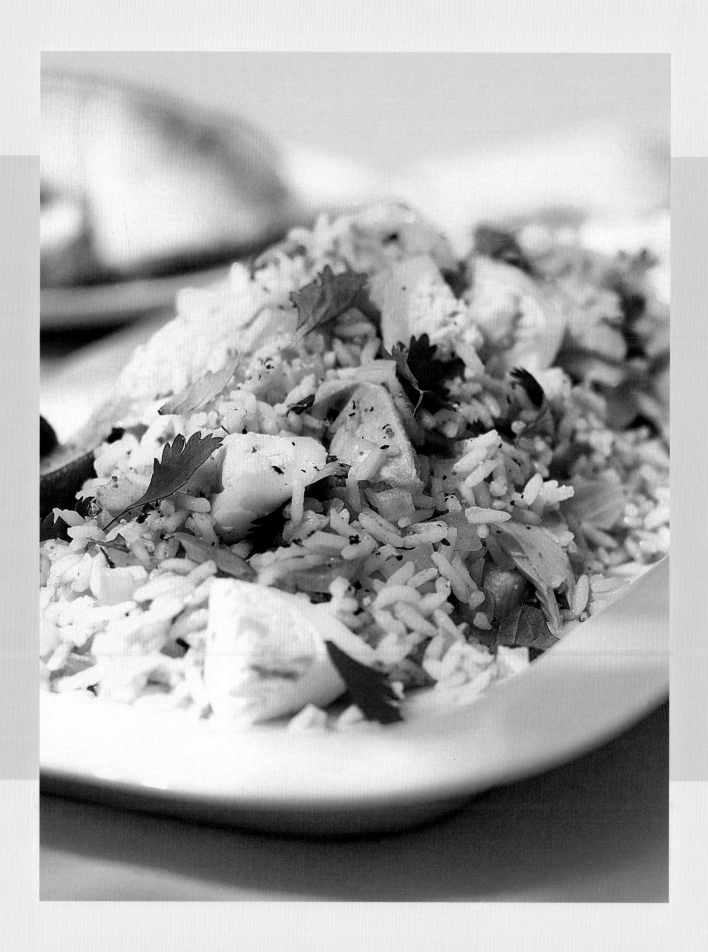

1

Breakfasts

OAT COOKIES WITH RAISINS & SOUR CHERRIES

Instead of buying expensive muesli bars, try these moist, fruity cookies, which can be warmed up in the oven or microwave. There is unlikely to be a healthier way to start your day.

115 g butter

85 g light brown sugar

115 g self-raising flour

Pinch of salt

140 g porridge oats or rolled oats

1 large egg, beaten

150 ml skimmed milk

115 g dried sour cherries

115 g raisins

Makes 25–30 cookies

1 Preheat the oven to 180° C, gas mark 4. In a large mixing bowl, cream the butter and sugar together, then mix in the flour, salt and oats.

2 Add the beaten egg and most of the milk until the mixture is stiff – you may not need to add all the milk. Mix thoroughly, and fold in the dried fruit. Give it a final mix.

3 Using a teaspoon, place walnut-size pieces onto a non-stick baking tray (the mixture spreads only slightly, so they do not need to be too far apart).

4 Bake in the oven for about 20 minutes or until golden brown.

HOME-MADE CRUNCHY MUESLI

This luxury muesli is a satisfying mix of sweet, golden apricots, sunflower seeds and crunchy chopped pecans in a rolled oat base. Serve with semi-skimmed milk, berries, slices of fresh fruit and a swirl of low-fat crème fraîche

350 g quick rolled oats

55 g roasted sunflower seeds

175 g seedless raisins

55 g chopped pecans

55 g 'ready-to-eat' dried apricots, chopped

Makes 14 servings

1 Mix all the ingredients together thoroughly, and transfer the muesli to an airtight container to store.

2 To serve, spoon into a serving bowl, pour over some semi-skimmed milk and add slices of your favourite fresh fruit and a creamy topping such as low-fat crème fraîche.

ALMOND & APPLE MUESLI

Replace the raisins with 150 g chopped dried apple slices and substitute 55 g of flaked almonds for the pecans. Mix the ingredients together as above.

APRICOT BRAN BREAKFAST MUFFINS

Muffins make a delicious treat for breakfast. These are very easy to make and are studded with sweet, golden apricots.

1 Soak the bran in the skimmed milk for 30 minutes. Meanwhile, preheat the oven to 200°C, gas mark 6.

2 Beat the egg, treacle, oil and sugar into the soaked bran, then sift the flour, baking powder, salt and bicarbonate of soda into the mixture. Add the apricots, and fold them in lightly but thoroughly, using a large spoon. If you prefer, 85 g of sultanas can be used in place of the apricots.

3 Spoon the mixture into 8 paper-lined bun or muffin tins and bake for 25 minutes or until they are cooked through. Serve warm. The sultana muffins can be split when still warm and served with reduced-sugar apricot jam.

55 g natural bran

150 ml skimmed milk

1 large egg, beaten

1 tablespoon black treacle

50 ml sunflower oil

55 g soft brown sugar

85 g plain wholemeal flour

½ teaspoon baking powder

Pinch each of salt and bicarbonate of soda

85 g dried apricots, soaked overnight, drained and finely chopped

Makes 8

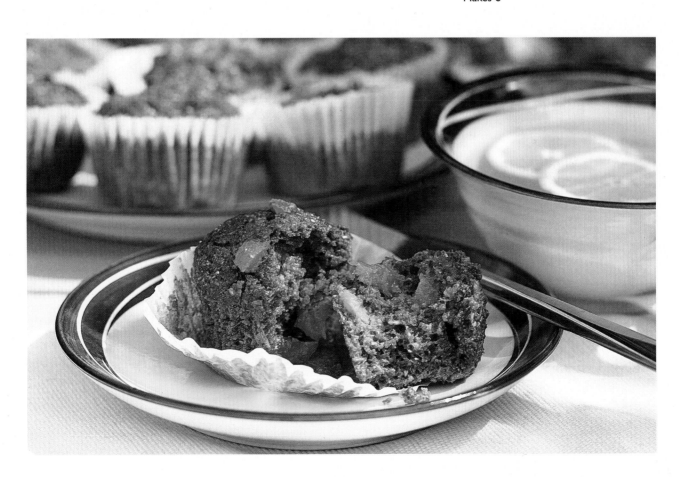

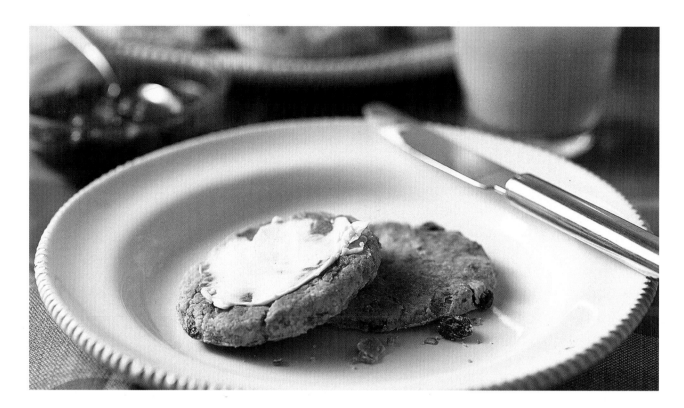

FRUITY BREAKFAST PANCAKES

55 g self-raising flour

55 g wholewheat flour

½ teaspoon baking powder

25 g caster sugar

Pinch ground cinnamon

55 g chilled sunflower margarine

25 g sultanas

Zest of 1 lemon, finely chopped

1 medium egg, beaten with 2 teaspoons skimmed milk

1 teaspoon sunflower oil

Makes 8

These breakfast pancakes are fragrant with cinnamon, lemon and juicy sultanas, though you can choose any mixture of dried fruit. They are traditionally cooked on a solid cast iron griddle, but if you don't have one, use a large heavy-based frying pan.

1 Sift the flours, baking powder, sugar and cinnamon into a large bowl, adding any bran that remains in the sieve.

2 Dice the margarine, and lightly rub it into the dry ingredients with your fingertips until the mixture resembles coarse breadcrumbs.

3 Stir in the dried fruit, add the lemon zest and fold in the egg and milk mixture, a little at a time, to make a soft dough.

4 Transfer to a lightly floured pastry board, and roll out to about 1 cm thick. With a 7 cm pastry cutter, cut the dough into rounds. Gather up any scraps and roll them out again until all the dough is used up.

5 Lightly grease the griddle or frying pan with half of the oil, and heat over a medium heat. Place 4 pancakes on the hot surface, and cook them for 2–3 minutes on each side, until they are browned and cooked through.

6 Grease the griddle or frying pan with the rest of the oil and cook the rest of the pancakes in the same way. Serve hot, with low-fat spread, if desired.

HONEY GRILLED GRAPEFRUIT WITH TOASTED SESAME SEEDS

Drizzled with honey, scattered with sesame seeds and grilled to perfection, your breakfast grapefruit is infused with sweet honey and nut flavours. If you don't have sesame seeds, sprinkle some wheatgerm or flaked almonds on top.

1. Using a sharp kitchen knife, cut a small piece from the bottom of each grapefruit half, so that the flat base of the fruit will sit comfortably on the rack of your grill pan.

2. Preheat the grill. Take a grapefruit or other 'saw-edged' knife and carefully cut around each grapefruit half, gently loosening the flesh from the skin. Then cut between the segments, so that they will be easy to spoon out.

3. Spoon the honey onto the top of each grapefruit half, pressing gently so that it oozes through the segments.

4. Arrange the grapefruit halves on the grill rack, and grill under a medium heat for about 2 minutes.

5. Sprinkle over the sesame seeds and grill for a further 30 seconds (no longer, or the seeds will burn). Serve immediately.

2 large pink grapefruit, halved, pips removed

40 g clear honey

15 g sesame seeds

Serves 4

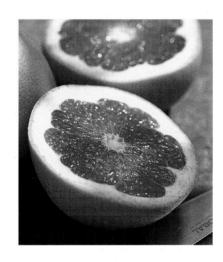

BANANA & MANGO YOGURT SMOOTHIE WITH WHEATGERM

Smoothies make a great start to your day, and taste utterly delicious. You can use different combinations of fruit, but make sure it is ripe.

1. Put the fruit into a blender or food processor, add the yogurt and skimmed milk and process for a few seconds until smooth.

2. Pour into 2 serving glasses and chill for at least 1 hour.

3. Mix the wheatgerm and honey together, and stir the mixture into the smoothie just before serving.

1 medium banana, peeled and chopped

1 medium ripe mango, peeled and diced

200 g low-fat natural yogurt

150 ml skimmed milk

FOR THE TOPPING

25 g wheatgerm

25 g clear honey

Serves 2

PAPAYA & STRAWBERRY SMOOTHIE

Mix a chopped ripe papaya with 150 g halved strawberries in a blender and then blend in the low-fat natural yogurt and skimmed milk as above. Scatter with passion fruit seeds before serving.

SCRAMBLED EGGS WITH SMOKED SALMON

4 medium eggs

Pinch of salt and black pepper

Good pinch red chilli powder

1 teaspoon sunflower oil

4 spring onions, sliced

1 red pepper, diced

115 g smoked salmon, sliced

Serves 4

This creamy mixture of egg and smoked salmon is quick and easy to prepare and the red pepper adds an interesting crunchy texture.

1 Beat the eggs with the seasoning and chilli powder.

2 Heat the oil and stir-fry the onions and peppers for a couple of minutes, until they have softened.

3 Pour the egg mixture over the onions and peppers. Stir continuously until the eggs are cooked through, but are still moist and creamy. Stir in the salmon, warm and serve immediately.

EGGS FLORENTINE

4 medium eggs

15 g butter

1 small onion, finely chopped

300 g babyleaf spinach

2 granary baps, halved

20 g cheddar cheese, finely grated

Salt and pepper, to taste

Serves 4

A light, balanced breakfast of poached egg on a bed of buttered spinach all piled onto thick granary bread – a perfect combination. Remember to cook the spinach lightly so as to preserve all the natural goodness as well as a bit of bite! You can use a tablespoon of olive oil instead of the butter if you like.

1 Poach the eggs until they are cooked but not runny.

2 Heat the butter in a non-stick pan. Add the onion and fry for 2-3 minutes.

3 Add the spinach and stir-fry until it has just wilted and the moisture has evaporated. Season to taste.

4 Toast the halved baps and lay them onto warmed plates. Smother the bap with the spinach and place a poached egg on top.

5 Finish with freshly ground black pepper and a little grated cheese.

SALMON KEDGEREE WITH FRESH CORIANDER

Kedgeree is the perfect dish for a lazy weekend breakfast or Sunday brunch. It is usually made with smoked haddock, but in this lighter version, the delicate flavour of salmon is highlighted with fragrant coriander. Serve it hot on triangles of toast.

1 Place the salmon fillets in a shallow pan with the water, wine, bay leaf, salt and pepper and bring to the boil.

2 Lower the heat and poach gently for 5 minutes. Remove from the heat and leave to cool in the cooking liquid.

3 Heat the oil in a large, heavy-based pan and gently fry the onion until softened but not browned. Stir in the curry powder and cook, stirring continuously, for a further minute. Add the rice, stir it thoroughly into the onion mixture, and put on one side.

4 Once the salmon is cool enough to handle, lift it from the cooking liquid with a slotted spoon. Flake the flesh, and remove any skin and bones.

5 Strain the cooking liquid into a measuring jug, and add enough water to make 568 ml. Pour this into the rice mixture, and bring it to the boil. Stir once, lower the heat and cook for about 12 minutes until the rice is tender and the liquid is absorbed.

6 Carefully fold in the salmon and eggs, and try not to break them up too much. Adjust the seasoning, if necessary, and serve hot, garnished with finely chopped fresh coriander.

TRADITIONAL KEDGEREE

Boil the rice in vegetable stock and plenty of water, drain and set aside. Poach 300g of smoked haddock in a shallow pan. Drain and flake the fish, removing any bones. Heat 1 tablespoon of corn oil and sauté 100 g sliced mushrooms and 1 finely chopped onion for about 5 minutes. Mix the cooked fish, rice, mushrooms and onions together. Add 100 g of boiled peas, 1 tablespoon of fresh lemon or lime juice and seasoning. Place the mixture in a covered oven-proof dish and bake for 15–20 minutes (170˚C, gas mark 3).

Ingredients
350 g salmon fillets
150 ml water
150 ml dry white wine
1 bay leaf
Salt and pepper, to taste
1 tablespoon sunflower oil
1 large onion, finely chopped
2 teaspoons curry powder
200 g easy-cook long-grain rice
2 medium eggs, hard-boiled and quartered
2 tablespoons finely chopped coriander, to garnish
Serves 4

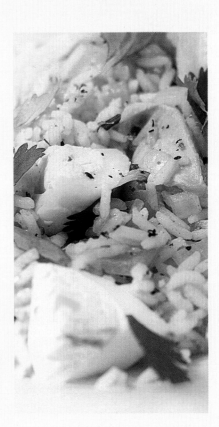

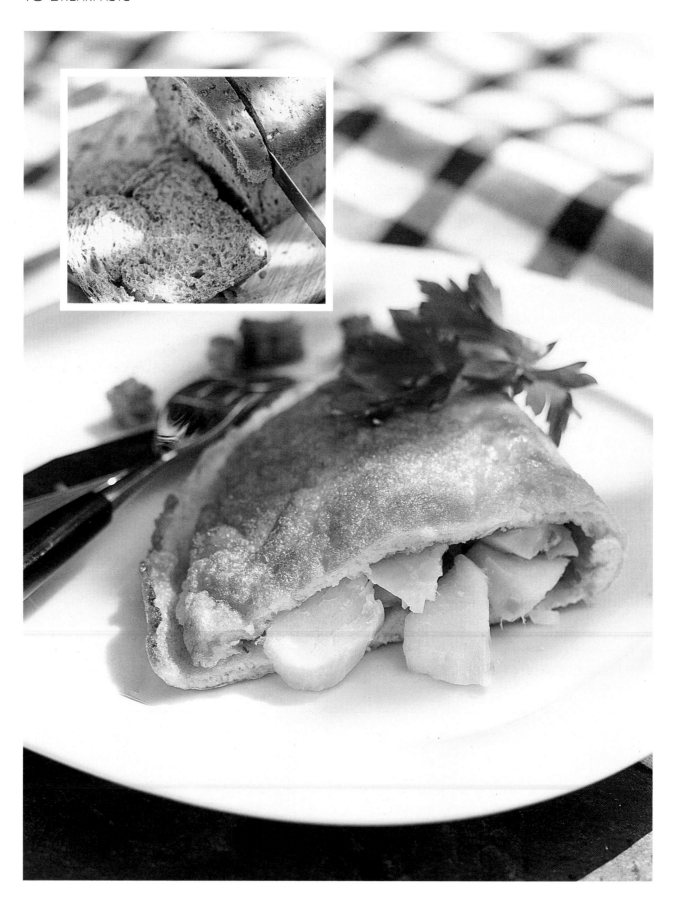

SMOKED HADDOCK SOUFFLÉ OMELETTE WITH CROÛTONS

This feathery light, melt-in-the-mouth omelette makes a special weekend brunch enough for two people. If you have guests, you can simply double the quantities, use a larger omelette pan and serve four.

1   Make the croûtons. Heat the oil in a large, heavy-based frying pan and fry the squares of bread on both sides until crisp. Drain on kitchen paper.

2   Put the fish in a pan with enough water to cover it. Bring it to the boil, lower the heat and poach gently for 5 minutes or until cooked through. Leave in the poaching liquid until cool enough to handle, lift it out of the cooking liquid with a slotted spoon and drain. Discard the liquid.

3   Beat the egg yolks in a large bowl and season with salt and pepper.

4   In another clean, dry, bowl, using a clean, dry, whisk, whip the whites until they stand up in soft peaks. Using a large metal spoon, fold them lightly but thoroughly into the beaten yolks.

5   Preheat the grill to high. Meanwhile, heat the butter or margarine in a 20 cm non-stick omelette pan, then pour in the egg mixture.

6   Cook over a moderate heat for 4–5 minutes, gently lifting the edges of the omelette with a spatula, so that the egg mixture runs underneath and the omelette cooks through.

7   Place the pan under the grill and cook the omelette for a further 2–3 minutes until the top is set.

8   Spoon the flaked haddock over one half of the omelette, then tilt the pan, and use a spatula to fold it in half.

9   Slide the omelette onto a warm plate and cut it in half. Scatter the top of the omelette with the croûtons and serve immediately.

175 g undyed smoked haddock fillet

FOR THE CROÛTONS

1 tablespoon sunflower oil

2 medium slices wholemeal bread from a large loaf (about 35 g each), cut into small squares

FOR THE OMELETTE

3 large eggs, separated

Salt and pepper, to taste

15 g butter or polyunsaturated margarine

Serves 2

WILD MUSHROOM TOASTS

400 g baby new potatoes, sliced (unpeeled)

1 teaspoon olive oil

Salt and pepper, to taste

FOR THE MUSHROOMS

1 tablespoon olive oil

4 medium shallots, chopped

450 g wild mushrooms

Spray oil

8 vine tomatoes, halved

3 tablespoons chopped fresh parsley

3 tablespoons chopped fresh chives

2 tablespoons half-fat crème fraîche

Salt and pepper, to taste

4 slices thick white bread

TO SERVE

1 tablespoon pine nuts

1 tablespoon fresh chopped chives

Serves 4

A mouth-watering breakfast, which has the freshness of wild mushrooms, flavoured with fresh parsley, shallots, chives and crème fraîche. The mushrooms are piled on top of layers of sliced potato and crusty white bread and are served with griddled vine tomatoes. A scattering of toasted pine nuts and chopped chives add the finishing touches.

1 Boil the potatoes until they are just cooked but still keep their shape. Drain, toss in a teaspoon of olive oil and season. Keep warm.

2 Heat a heavy-based frying pan and toast the pine nuts over a low heat, stirring continuously. Remove the pine nuts from heat, set them to one side and allow them to cool.

3 Meanwhile, heat the oil in a non-stick pan and fry the shallots to soften.

4 Stir in the mushrooms and fry gently for 4–5 minutes.

5 Meanwhile, heat a few sprays of oil in a griddle pan. Gently place the tomatoes, skin side up in the pan. Cook on both sides till the tomatoes are charred and soft, yet still in shape. Reserve until ready to use.

6 Whilst the tomatoes are cooking, add the fresh parsley and chives to the mushrooms. Stir in the crème fraîche, season to taste and heat through.

7 Toast the bread lightly and place each slice onto a warmed plate. Spoon a layer of the sliced potatoes on top.

8 Pile the mushrooms onto the potatoes and top with a sprinkling of toasted pine nuts and chopped chives.

9 Add the griddled tomatoes to the plate and serve immediately while everything is hot.

POTATO CAKES

If you have any leftover mashed potato, transform it into a tasty treat. These pancakes can be served with lean grilled bacon and tomatoes, cold ham with grated cheese melted over the top, baked beans or a scraping of butter.

280 g cooked potato, mashed with a little skimmed milk

55 g fine oatmeal

40 g plain flour (plus extra for dusting)

Pinch of salt

Makes 12

1 Place all the ingredients in a large mixing bowl and mix together with your hands to make a pliable dough.

2 Take a third of the mixture, place it on a lightly floured surface and roll into a thin circle, about 15–18 cm in diameter.

3 Prick the dough all over with a fork, and cut it into 4 triangles.

4 Heat a heavy-based frying pan or griddle until it is very hot. Do not add any fat. Place the 4 cakes on the hot surface, and cook for about 3 minutes on each side until they are golden brown.

5 Keep the finished potato cakes warm by wrapping them in a clean tea towel and put them to one side while you make the rest. Cook the remaining 2 batches as before, and serve hot.

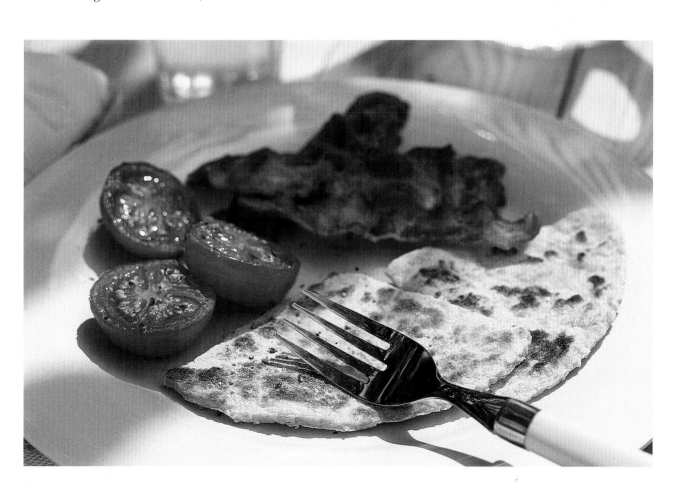

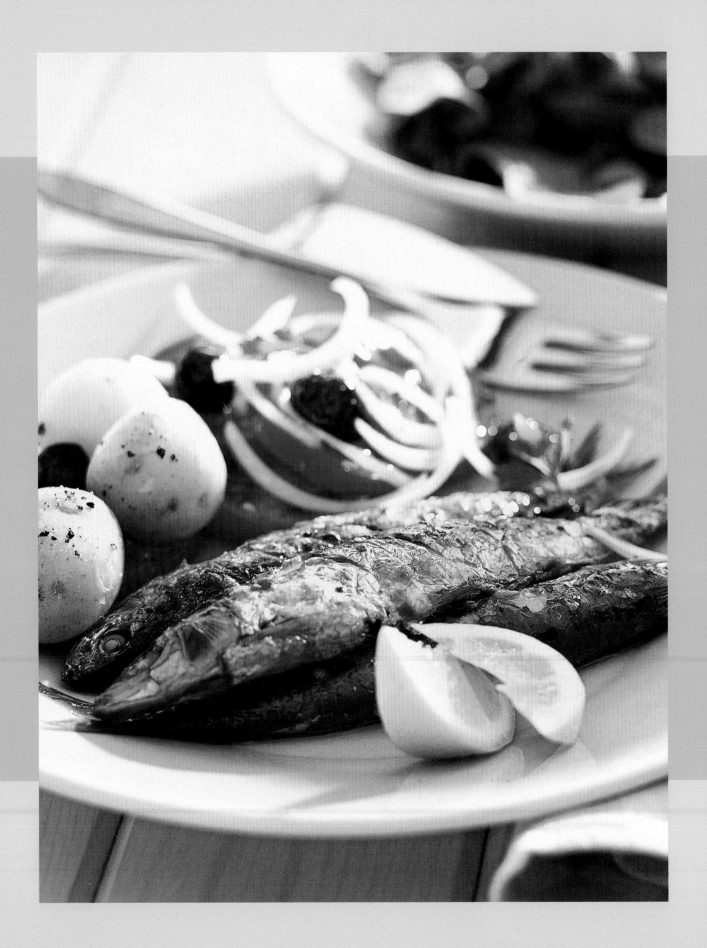

Light Meals & Snacks

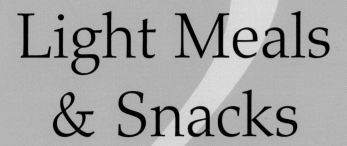

PRAWN & APPLE PITTA POCKETS

6 crab sticks, diced

100 g cooked prawns

1 large apple, cored and diced

2 tablespoons low-fat mild mustard dressing

4 mini pitta breads

4 crisp lettuce leaves, shredded

Serves 4

Pitta bread opens up into a convenient pocket that can be generously filled to make a light but satisfying meal. Try this seafood version – it's great for picnics and packed lunches.

1 In a bowl, mix the crab sticks, prawns, apple and dressing together. If you prefer, you can make Tuna & Apple Pitta Pockets by substituting the prawns with 100 g (drained weight) tuna canned in brine.

2 Fill the pittas with some of the lettuce and top with the seafood mix.

LAYERED MEDITERRANEAN SANDWICH

175 g ciabatta loaf (a thin rectangular one is best)

2 teaspoons fat-free vinaigrette

2 medium beef tomatoes, sliced

2 peppers (one each of red and yellow), roasted and sliced

115 g buffalo mozzarella

5 black olives, stones removed

Few fresh basil leaves

Salt and pepper, to taste

Serves 4

This sandwich is infused with sunny, luscious Mediterranean flavours. It also improves with keeping for up to six hours, so it's ideal to take to work or as part of a picnic lunch. You can vary the flavour of your sandwich depending on what ingredients you have available. Experiment with combinations of tuna, roasted aubergines, boiled egg slices, rocket leaves, sliced red onions, anchovy fillets or grated carrot.

1 Cut the loaf in half horizontally and sprinkle some vinaigrette dressing over both sides of the loaf.

2 Layer the rest of the ingredients onto one half of the loaf, season with salt and pepper, and sprinkle over the remainder of the vinaigrette.

3 Place the other half of the loaf on top and wrap the sandwich tightly in aluminium foil or cling film.

4 Store in the refrigerator – place the sandwich underneath a heavy object to flatten it until ready to serve.

5 Unwrap and cut into slices.

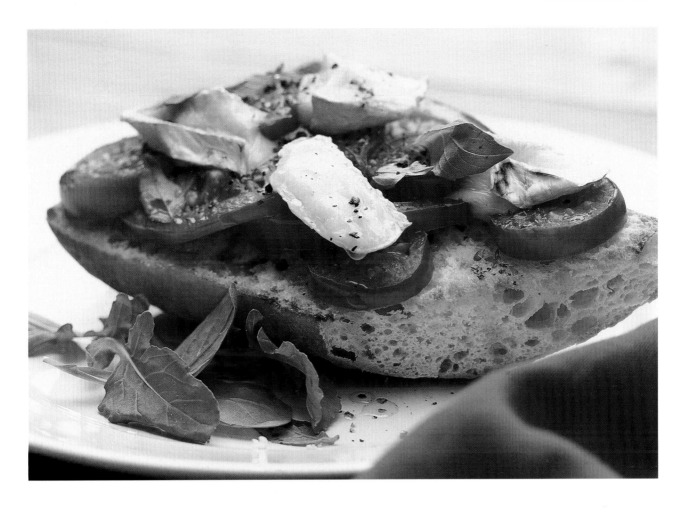

GOAT'S CHEESE, TOMATO & CIABATTA GRILL

Simplicity itself, this grilled sandwich is ideal for a light lunch or supper. Use the ripest tomatoes you can find, as their sweetness will provide a delicious contrast to the sharpness of the goat's cheese. It is also very good made with mozzarella cheese, using the same quantities.

1 Preheat the grill to medium. Arrange the ciabatta slices on the grill tray, and drizzle with the olive oil.

2 Top with the sliced tomatoes, sprinkle them with the herbs, then grill for about 3 minutes or until the tomatoes are soft and pulpy.

3 Add the cheese slices, season well, and grill for a further 3–4 minutes.

4 Serve with the mixed salad leaves, garnished with sprigs of fresh basil.

4 x 50 g slices ciabatta bread

2 teaspoons extra virgin olive oil

4 small vine tomatoes, sliced

1 teaspoon Herbes de Provence

115 g goat's cheese, thinly sliced

Salt and pepper, to taste

50 g mixed salad leaves, to serve

4 small sprigs fresh basil, to garnish

Serves 2

PORTUGUESE SARDINE SALAD

1 kg ready-prepared sardines (thawed if frozen)

Pinch coarse sea salt

1 tablespoon lemon juice

1 teaspoon piri-piri or other hot pepper sauce

700 g new potatoes in their skins

FOR THE SALAD

6 medium tomatoes, sliced

1 small onion, thinly sliced

50 g black olives

2 tablespoons olive oil

2 teaspoons white wine vinegar

Salt and pepper, to taste

Serves 6

Fresh sardines are absolutely delicious – ask the fishmonger to clean and gut them. Alternatively, buy them frozen and ready-prepared. The traditional Portuguese way of serving them is with plain boiled potatoes and a simple salad of tomatoes, onion and black olives.

1 Preheat the grill to high. Make 2 or 3 slits in the plumpest part of each sardine using a sharp knife.

2 Mix together the sea salt, lemon juice and hot sauce and rub into the slits.

3 Cook the sardines under a hot grill for 5–8 minutes each side – the grilling time will depend on their size.

4 While the sardines are cooking, boil and drain the potatoes.

5 Make the salad. Put the tomatoes, onion slices and olives in a bowl. To make the dressing, put the olive oil, wine vinegar and seasoning in a screw top jar, and shake thoroughly.

6 Serve the sardines with the potatoes, and the salad tossed in the dressing on the side.

TUNA & DILL SALAD WITH VEGETABLE CRUDITÉS

200 g canned tuna in brine, drained

4 tablespoons fat-free vinaigrette dressing

125 ml low-fat natural yogurt

15 g fresh dill, finely chopped

Salt and pepper, to taste

20 cm stick cucumber, cut into strips

3 medium carrots, cut into sticks

3 celery sticks, cut into 8 cm pieces

2 red peppers, cut into strips

Serves 4

These juicy, crunchy vegetable strips make a piquant and colourful contrast to the tuna salad which is scented with the delicious aniseed flavour of fresh dill. A perfect summer snack.

1 Prepare the tuna dip by mixing together the tuna, vinaigrette dressing, low-fat yogurt, dill and seasoning.

2 Chill the tuna in the refrigerator and serve with the fresh vegetable strips.

AVOCADO WITH WARM SHREDDED CHICKEN & WALNUT SALAD

Here's something special – a light but luscious meal that will gratify your tastebuds. The flavours of the avocados and walnuts combine perfectly with the chicken, and this is ideal for lunch or supper.

1 Put the avocado slices into a bowl with the lemon juice and mix gently.

2 Heat the olive oil in a wok or non-stick frying pan (a wok is better), and stir-fry the shredded chicken for 3–4 minutes or until it is cooked through.

3 Add the pimento slices and stir-fry for 1 further minute.

4 Remove from the heat, then drain the lemon juice from the avocados, and stir it into the chicken. Mix in the seasoning, mustard and sugar.

5 Arrange the avocado slices onto 4 serving plates, add the chicken salad and serve garnished with the walnuts.

4 avocados, peeled, stoned and sliced

2 tablespoons lemon juice

FOR THE SALAD

2 tablespoons extra virgin olive oil

3 x 150 g skinless and boneless chicken breasts, finely shredded

100 g canned red pimento, drained and finely sliced

Salt and pepper, to taste

2 teaspoons French mustard

1 teaspoon caster sugar

50 g chopped walnuts, to garnish

Serves 4

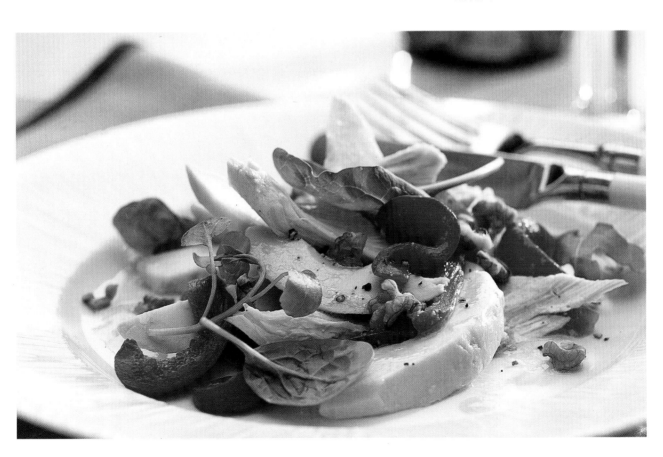

WARM LENTILS & CHILLI BEANS WITH SMOKED BACON

225 g Puy lentils

225 g canned red kidney beans, drained

Salt and pepper, to taste

½ teaspoon hot pepper sauce (or to taste)

1 tablespoon olive oil

1 medium onion, finely chopped

175 g lean, smoked bacon, diced

100 g half-fat crème fraîche and a sprinkling hot paprika, to garnish

Serves 4

This is best made with green Puy lentils – they're available from large supermarkets. However, if you can't get them, use any lentils, and follow the packet instructions for cooking times. This is a great dish for people with diabetes, as the beans and lentils allow blood glucose to rise slowly.

1 Cook the lentils according to the packet instructions – if you are using Puy lentils, this should take about 35 minutes.

2 Place the lentils in a bowl, and add the drained kidney beans, seasoning and hot pepper sauce. Mix together thoroughly.

3 Heat the oil in a non-stick heavy-based frying pan, and gently sauté the onion for 2–3 minutes until softened but not browned.

4 Add the smoked bacon and cook, stirring, for a further 3 minutes.

5 Add the bacon and onions to the lentil and bean mixture, mix thoroughly and serve garnished with crème fraîche and a sprinkling of hot paprika.

BEAN & VEGETABLE STEW

1 tablespoon. olive oil

2 garlic cloves, crushed

1 medium onion, chopped

1 green pepper, diced

300 g sweet potatoes, peeled and chopped into cubes

4 large tomatoes, chopped

1 teaspoon dried mixed herbs

Salt and pepper, to taste

225 g frozen whole green beans, defrosted

400 g can red kidney beans

3 tablespoons freshly chopped parsley

Serves 4

A warming stew of fresh vegetables with a mix of green beans and red kidney beans. The sweet potato makes this into a delightfully unusual dish.

1 Heat the oil in a large pan with a lid. Fry the garlic, onion and green pepper until the have softened.

2 Add the sweet potato, tomatoes, herbs and seasoning. Stir well, cover and cook for 20-25 minutes until the sweet potato is cooked but not mushy.

3 Add the green beans and the kidney beans to the potato stew, stir and allow to cook for a few more minutes.

4 When cooked, adjust the seasoning and top with parsley.

TUSCAN BREAD SALAD WITH RED ONION & MOZZARELLA

This is a version of a traditional Italian peasant snack, and is an ideal way of using up stale bread. It has to be the right kind of bread, though – a coarse, dense-textured loaf is just what you need. Ciabatta is a good choice, and it should be at least 3 or 4 days old.

1 Sprinkle the bread on both sides with just enough water to moisten it.

2 Place the slices on individual serving plates and sprinkle the wine vinegar over one side only. Season with salt and pepper.

3 Arrange layers of vegetables and cheese on each slice of bread, drizzle with the olive oil, and serve garnished with sprigs of fresh basil.

4 x 50 g slices stale ciabatta

25 ml red wine vinegar

Salt and pepper, to taste

6 medium ripe tomatoes, sliced

2 small red onions, thinly sliced

1 stick celery, including leaves, thinly sliced

175 g mozzarella cheese, thinly sliced

3 tablespoons extra virgin olive oil

4 small sprigs basil, to garnish

Serves 4

SAVOURY POPCORN SNACK

Here's a scrumptious, deliciously healthy snack that won't send your blood sugar soaring. Popcorn is made from dried sweetcorn, and it's packed with slowly absorbed fibre. By making it yourself, you can make sure it's low-fat.

1 Heat a heavy-based non-stick pan with a tight-fitting lid until it is very hot. Pour in the oil and keep the heat turned up high.

2 Add the corn then cover with the lid. The corn will start to pop and bounce off the lid. Remove the pan from the heat immediately the popping stops.

3 Season with a little salt and as much lemon juice as you like, and serve.

1 teaspoon corn oil

2 heaped tablespoons popping corn

Pinch salt

Fresh lemon juice, to taste

Serves 4

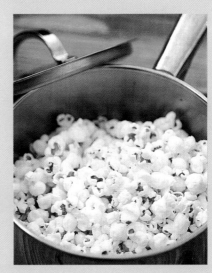

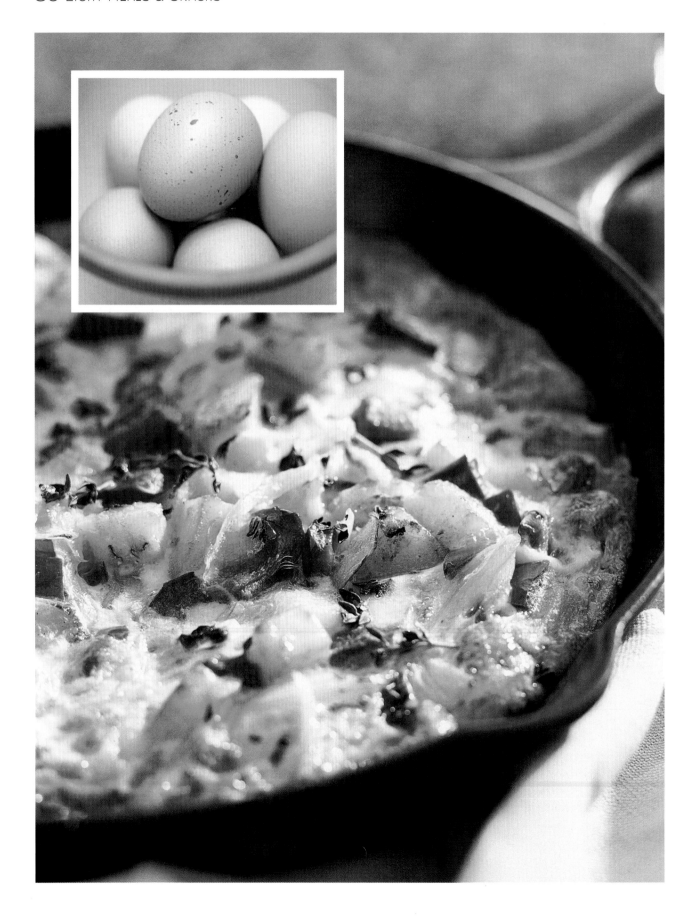

POTATO, RED PEPPER & ONION FRITTATA

This typical Italian-style omelette is flavoured with tasty onion and peppers. It is equally delicious served hot, warm, or cold and makes a great picnic dish.

1 Preheat the grill to high. Boil the diced potatoes in lightly salted water for 5 minutes or until they are just tender. Drain them well.

2 Heat the oil in a large, heavy-based, non-stick frying pan and gently sauté the onion for 3–4 minutes until it is softened but not browned.

3 Add the cooked potato and red pepper, increase the heat slightly and cook for a further 2–3 minutes, stirring gently, until the potatoes turn golden.

4 Beat the eggs with the water, season to taste, then mix in the herbs.

5 Pour the eggs evenly over the vegetables in the pan and cook over a medium heat for 2–3 minutes until the base is nicely browned.

6 Transfer the pan to the grill and cook for a further 2 minutes or until the top is set and a deep golden brown. Serve in wedges.

175 g potatoes, peeled and diced

1 tablespoon olive oil

1 medium onion, peeled and thinly sliced

1 red pepper, deseeded, cored and diced

4 large eggs

1 tablespoon cold water

Salt and pepper, to taste

1 teaspoon chopped fresh thyme or oregano

Serves 4

VEGETABLE GRATIN

Fast and tasty, this can be an accompaniment or served as a light meal with warm French crusty bread.

1 Steam the carrots in a little boiling water for about 3 minutes.

2 Add the cauliflower, broccoli and peas, cover and cook until the vegetables are just tender. Drain and put the vegetables in a large, lightly greased flameproof dish, cover and keep warm.

3 Make up the cheese sauce as directed on the packet. Stir in the mustard and the seasoning. Preheat the grill to medium.

4 Pour the sauce over the vegetables and mix gently. Top with the grated cheese and tomato slices.

5 Grill under medium heat for 5 minutes. Serve immediately.

3 medium carrots, peeled and sliced

1 medium cauliflower, divided into florets

115 g broccoli florets

100 g frozen petit pois

40 g packet instant cheese sauce mix

1 teaspoon Dijon mustard

Salt and coarsely ground pepper

2 tablespoons finely grated cheddar cheese

2 vine tomatoes, sliced lengthways

Serves 4

PIZZA WITH THREE-COLOURED PEPPERS & BEANS

FOR THE BASE

115 g strong plain white flour

115 g wholemeal flour

1 teaspoon easy-blend yeast

¼ teaspoon salt

150 ml lukewarm water

1 tablespoon sunflower oil

FOR THE TOPPING

2 teaspoons olive oil

1 medium red onion, roughly chopped

1 red pepper, deseeded, cored and sliced

1 yellow pepper, deseeded, cored and sliced

1 green pepper, deseeded, cored and sliced

1 x 400 g can red kidney beans, rinsed and drained

Salt and pepper, to taste

2 tablespoons tomato pureé

1 x 400 g can chopped tomatoes with garlic

115 g grated mozzarella cheese

1 x 15 g pack fresh basil leaves, torn

Serves 4

This is a gloriously colourful pizza, and has lots of slowly absorbed fibre to keep your blood sugar steady. You could buy the base ready-made, of course, and just use the topping. However, it's much nicer to cook your own – then you'll know how pizza really should taste.

1   Preheat the oven to 220°C, gas mark 7. Sift the white and wholemeal flours into a large bowl, then stir in the yeast and salt.

2   Make a well in the centre of the flour mixture, and gradually mix in the water and oil to form a soft dough.

3   Transfer the dough to a lightly-floured board, and knead it for about 10 minutes until it is smooth and elastic.

4   Return the dough to the bowl (cleaned, if necessary), cover with a tea towel and leave it to stand in a warm place for about 1 hour or until the dough has doubled in size.

5   While the dough is rising, heat the oil for the topping in a heavy-based non-stick pan, and stir-fry the onion and peppers for 3 minutes until they are soft but not browned.

6   Add the kidney beans and season to taste. Remove the pan from the heat and put it on one side.

7   Roll out the risen dough into a large circle, about 15-18 inches in diameter. Place it on a large, oiled, baking sheet or an oiled pizza pan.

8   Cover the pizza base with tomato purée, then spread over the chopped tomatoes. Top with the cooked vegetables, then sprinkle over the grated mozzarella and basil leaves.

9   Bake near the top of the oven for 25-30 minutes until the cheese is golden and bubbling. Serve immediately.

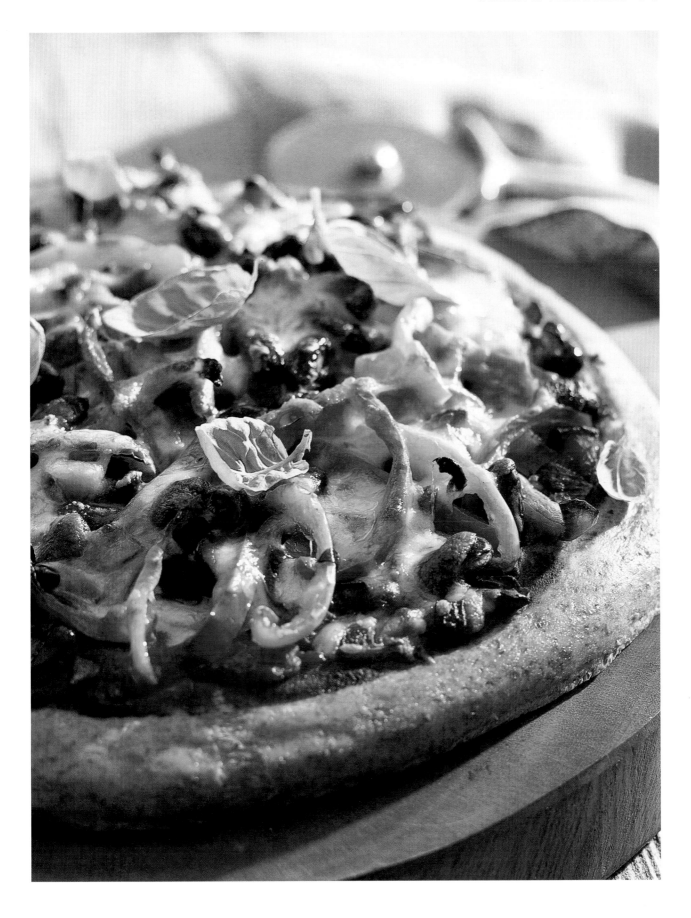

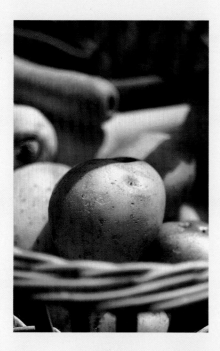

4 x 225 g baking potatoes

1 tablespoon sunflower oil

Serves 4

FILLED JACKET POTATOES

Jacket-baked potatoes are cosy and comforting – a true family favourite. They're also a boon to those with diabetes – the starchy carbohydrate they contain, coupled with the fibre in the skin make them especially nutritious. Traditional oven-baked potatoes are unbeatable, and you can ring the changes with the filling of your choice.

1 Preheat the oven to 200°C, gas mark 6.

2 Scrub the potatoes well and, while they are still damp, prick them in several places with a fork. Then rub them all over with the oil.

3 Bake the potatoes in the centre of the oven for about 1 hour 15 minutes, or until the skins are nice and crisp and the centres cooked through.

4 Remove them from oven. When the potatoes are cool enough to handle, cut them in half lengthways, and carefully scoop out most of the flesh into a bowl, leaving the skins intact.

5 Mix the cooked potato with your choice of the following fillings, and proceed as instructed for each filling method.

AVOCADO WITH PRAWNS
Scoop out the flesh of a large, ripe avocado into a bowl, and beat in 25 g half-fat crème fraîche. Stir in ½ teaspoon hot pepper sauce and 100 g cooked peeled prawns. Mix together with the cooked potato flesh, pile the mixture back into the potato shells, and return to the oven for 5 minutes before serving.

TUNA TRICOLOR
Mix 115 g (drained weight) tuna canned in brine with the cooked potato, season to taste and spoon into the potato shells. Return the potatoes to the oven and re-heat for 5 minutes. Meanwhile, prepare the topping. Mix together 50 g each of diced red and green pepper, 50 g sweetcorn kernels with 2 tablespoons reduced-calorie mayonnaise. Pile on top of the potatoes before serving.

SMOKED HAM WITH PESTO SAUCE
Make half the quantity of pesto sauce (see page 52) and stir it into the bowl of cooked potato. Add 100 g diced lean smoked ham and mix thoroughly. Pile the mixture back into the potato shells and top with 25 g Parmesan cheese shavings (use a potato peeler). Return to the oven for 5 minutes before serving.

BAKED CHEESY TRIANGLES

Quick cheese on toast can be made quite memorable with a few tasty additions. Serve these with a simple lettuce and cherry tomato salad or with the baked tomato and olive salad on page 81.

8 slices bread, with crusts removed

100 g reduced-fat cheddar cheese, grated

2 tablespoons freshly chopped parsley

1 medium egg, beaten

150 ml semi-skimmed milk

Good pinch of dried Herbes de Provence

Coarse black pepper

Serves 4

1 Preheat the oven to 180°C, gas mark 4.

2 Cover 4 of the slices of bread with the cheese and the parsley, then place the remaining slices of bread on top.

3 Cut each sandwich into 4 triangles and place in a shallow, lightly greased ovenproof dish.

4 Whisk the egg and the milk together with the herbs and pepper.

5 Pour the egg and herb mixture over the sandwiches and bake in the oven for 15 minutes until golden brown.

STUFFED PEPPERS

The traditional recipe for stuffed peppers can take around 40 minutes in the oven, not including preparation time for the rice filling. This method takes a less conventional but easy short-cut. The peppers cook in boiling water while you prepare the filling, so no time is wasted. Use this recipe for left-overs too. Serve with red cabbage coleslaw (see page 83) and extra bread.

4 red peppers

2 teaspoons corn oil

1 medium onion, finely chopped

2 cloves garlic, crushed

115 g frozen peas

115 g frozen sweetcorn

1 teaspoon dried mixed herbs

Salt and black pepper

2 tablespoons fresh parsley, chopped

115 g long grain rice, boiled

30 g reduced-fat cheddar cheese

Serves 4

1 Cut a circle round the stem end of each pepper and remove the seeds. Put this circle back onto the peppers to form a lid. Place the peppers upright in a saucepan half-filled with boiling water. Bring this back to the boil, cover and cook for 5-8 minutes to soften.

2 Meanwhile, heat the oil in a non-stick pan. Add the onion and garlic and fry over a gentle heat until the onion is softened.

3 Add the peas, sweetcorn and seasoning to the pan with a few tablespoons of hot water. Cover with a tight-fitting lid and cook the vegetables over a high heat for a few minutes.

4 Add the parsley and rice to the vegetables and stir gently.

5 Spoon the rice mixture into the peppers, sprinkle with grated cheese and cover with the pepper "lids". Serve hot.

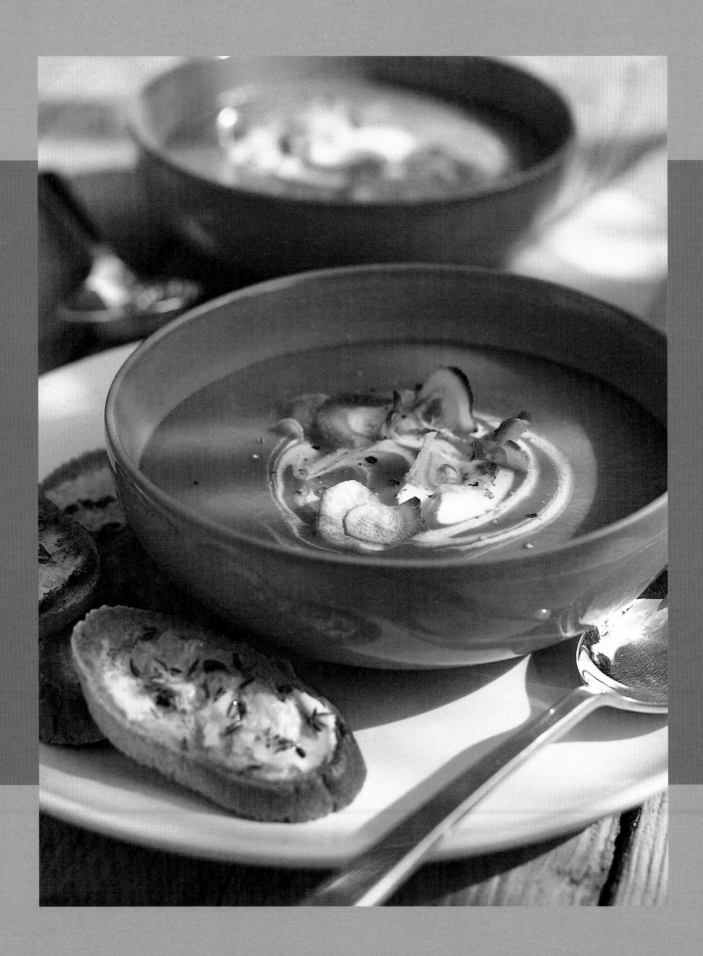

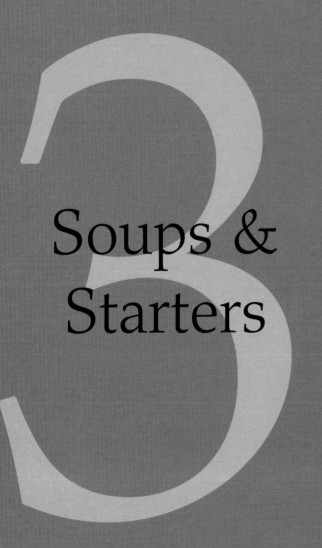

Soups & Starters

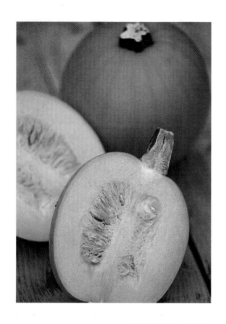

PUMPKIN SOUP WITH ROAST PARSNIP CRISPS

The brilliant golden flesh of pumpkin makes a creamy, appetising soup simply bursting with enticing garlic and ginger aromas. Choose small pumpkins, as they have more flesh and a better taste. This is also delicious with hot garlic bread on a chilly day.

1 Preheat the oven to 200°C, gas mark 6. Cut the pumpkin flesh into 5 cm chunks, and put them into an ovenproof dish with the ginger. Roast in the oven for 20 minutes.

2 Meanwhile prepare the crisps. Using a pastry brush, coat the slices of parsnip with corn oil, and lay them on an baking tray.

3 Roast the parsnip slices for 20 minutes in the oven, until they are crisp and golden, then set aside.

4 Make the soup. In a large pan, heat the oil and gently cook the onion and crushed garlic until soft.

5 Add the roasted pumpkin and ginger and pour in the vegetable stock. Bring to the boil and simmer gently for 15 minutes.

6 Pour the mixture into a blender and liquidise for about 1–2 minutes until it is smooth and creamy. Return the soup to the pan, and bring it back to the boil. Stir in the yogurt and adjust the seasoning.

7 Ladle into heated bowls and sprinkle with the parsnip crisps for garnish.

FOR THE SOUP

I kg pumpkin (about 750 g flesh peeled and deseeded)

25 g fresh root ginger, peeled

2 teaspoons corn oil

I medium onion, peeled and finely chopped

2 cloves garlic, peeled and crushed

750 ml vegetable stock

150 g low-fat natural yogurt

FOR THE CRISPS

3 medium parsnips, peeled and finely sliced

2 teaspoons corn oil

Serves 4–6

SWEET POTATO SOUP WITH CASSAVA CRISPS

Use 1 kg of chopped sweet potato and roast with a stick of cinnamon and a bay leaf. Follow the rest of the recipe as above. To make the crisps, finely slice 200 g of fresh peeled cassava and roast until crisp and browned.

BEAN & PASTA SOUP WITH BASIL

This is a deeply satisfying, rustic, Italian-style soup, packed full of hearty vegetables, beans and noodles. It makes a good, wholesome lunch served with warm, crusty bread.

1 Drain the tomatoes from the can, setting aside the juice for later.

2 In a large pan, heat the oil and cook the onion until soft. Add the stock, reduce the heat to low, cover and simmer for 5 minutes.

3 Add the green beans, courgettes and the reserved juice from the tomatoes. Season to taste, then simmer for 30 minutes.

4 Stir in the vermicelli and haricot beans. Simmer for a further 10 minutes.

5 Mix the pesto and tomatoes together and add to the soup. Bring it back to the boil, then serve immediately, sprinkled with the basil leaves.

115 g canned peeled tomatoes

1 tablespoon olive oil

1 medium onion, thinly sliced

1 litre chicken stock

125 g fresh green beans, cut into 1 cm lengths

2 small courgettes, diced

Salt and pepper, to taste

55 g vermicelli pasta

200 g white haricot beans, canned or pre-cooked according to the packet instructions

100 g pesto sauce

Few fresh basil leaves, to garnish

Serves 4–6

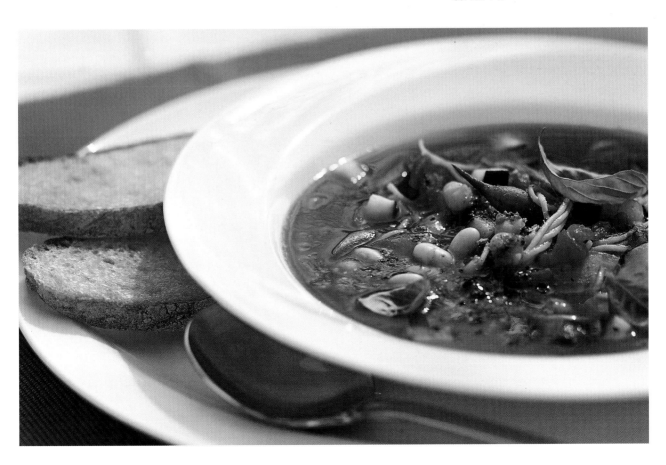

Red Lentil Soup

1 medium ham hock

1 litre water

450 g swede, peeled and cut into 6 cm chunks

2 medium carrots, grated

225 g red lentils, washed

Serves 4–6

This classic dish is a perfect marriage of earthy lentils with fragrant ham, and is popular with all the family. Lentils are highly effective at slowing down the rise in your blood sugar, so they are an excellent choice for diabetics.

1 In a large soup pan, cover the ham hock with the water and boil for 1 hour.

2 Add the swede, carrot and lentils and simmer for 30 minutes. Remove the ham pieces and the swede, and either keep them warm to eat as a main course, or put them in the refrigerator to use for another meal.

3 Let the soup cool slightly, then pour it into a blender and liquidise for about 1 minute, adding some more water if it is too thick.

4 Reheat thoroughly before serving.

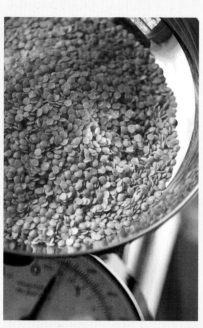

LENTIL & VEGETABLE SOUP
Omit the ham and water and substitute a good quality vegetable stock instead. This will shorten the preparation and cooking time to only 45 minutes. Use 180 g red lentils and simmer them with 2 sticks of chopped celery, 115g peeled chopped potato and the other vegetables as above. Garnish with a swirl of low-fat yogurt and a sprinkle of curry powder.

ROASTED RED PEPPER & LENTIL SOUP
Roast 2 red peppers under a preheated grill until they become slightly charred. Chop the peppers and add to the swede and lentil mixture. Continue as above.

Spinach & Onion Soup

1 tablespoon vegetable oil

2 medium onions, thinly sliced

900 ml vegetable stock

1 bay leaf

Salt and pepper

150 ml white wine

300 g baby leaf spinach

Serves 4

There is something satisfying about homemade soup! This recipe makes an ideal starter for any dinner party.

1 Heat the oil in a saucepan and fry the onions for about 5-8 minutes over a low heat, until they have softened.

2 Pour in the stock and bring to the boil. Add the bay leaf and the seasoning. Cover and simmer for 10 minutes.

3 Pour in the wine and add the spinach. Continue to cook, but only until the spinach has wilted slightly.

4 Remove the bay leaf and serve hot.

FISH & POTATO SOUP

This is a delicately flavoured soup, suffused with lovely smoky aromas from the fish. Be careful that you don't over-cook it — the fish and potatoes should have a slightly firm texture.

1 Put the the haddock in a large saucepan, add the water and cook over a low heat for 15 minutes.

2 Remove the fish from the water, roughly flake it and set it aside.

3 Add the onions, white pepper and potatoes to the remaining stock, then cover and cook over medium heat for 20 minutes.

4 Remove the pan from the heat, mash the potatoes in the pan, leaving a few chunky pieces for texture. Return the pan to a low heat heat, pour in the milk and add the flaked fish.

5 Simmer for 1 minute, season with the salt (if needed) and serve immediately, sprinkled with the chopped parsley.

450 g naturally smoked haddock
300 ml water
2 large onions, finely chopped
½ teaspoon white pepper
450 g potatoes, peeled and sliced
425 ml semi-skimmed milk
Pinch of salt
2 tablespoons finely chopped parsley, to garnish
Serves 4–6

PRAWN CHOWDER

Use only 250 g smoked haddock and add 225 g sweetcorn to the onions and potatoes and cook as above. After mashing the potatoes, return the mixture to the pan with 200 g cooked peeled prawns.

GARLIC BREAD

Commercially made garlic bread is often high in fat, but this easy version will help you to keep your weight on an even keel. It makes a wonderfully fragrant accompaniment to home-made soups

1 Preheat the grill to medium. Cut the French bread into 8 diagonal slices, place them under the grill and toast the slices on one side.

2 Mix the spread, garlic and thyme together. Spread the garlic mixture evenly over the untoasted side of the bread slices.

3 Arrange the slices of bread on the grill rack, flavoured side up, and grill until lightly browned. Serve immediately.

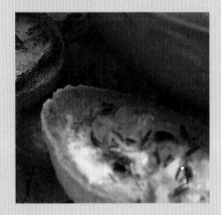

20 cm stick of French bread
55 g low-fat spread
1 clove garlic, crushed, or 1 teaspoon ready-made garlic paste
1 teaspoon finely chopped fresh thyme
Serves 4

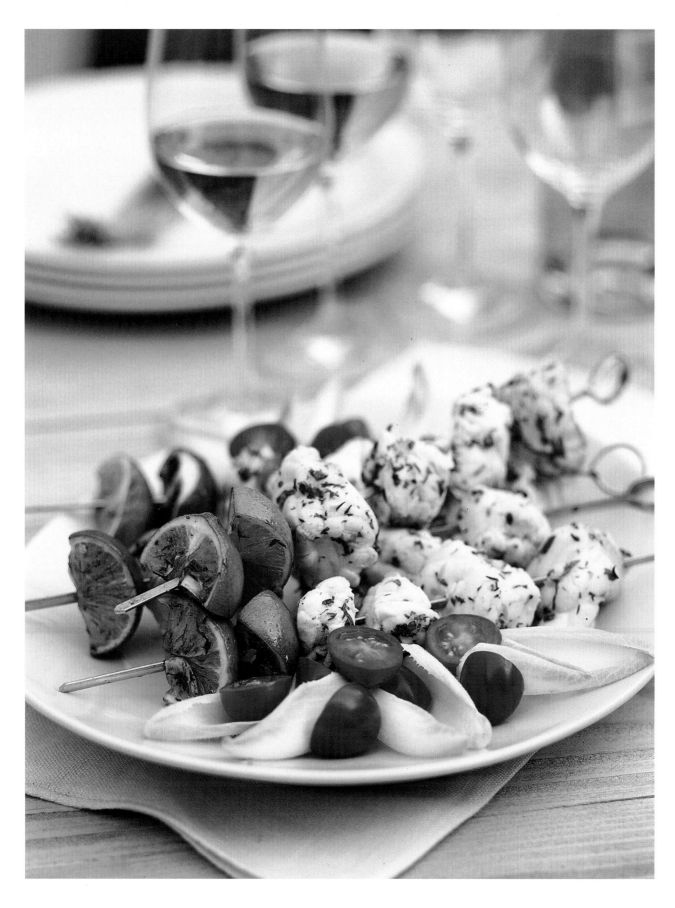

GARLIC PRAWNS

Tiger prawns are ideal for this dish as they are firm, plump, and full of briny juices. Serve them sizzling hot, and have plenty of crusty bread on hand to soak up the garlic-scented sauce.

1 Preheat the oven to 200°C, gas mark 6. Put the olive oil and garlic in a large, shallow ovenproof dish and heat in the oven for 2–3 minutes. You need to watch carefully so that the garlic does not start to brown.

2 Add the prawns, and roll them in the hot oil until they are completely coated. Return them to the oven and bake for a further 3 minutes until they are pink and cooked through.

3 Serve immediately, sprinkled with freshly chopped parsley. Served accompanied by lemon wedges for squeezing.

1 tablespoon olive oil

2 cloves garlic, peeled and thinly sliced

225 g large raw prawns (such as tiger prawns), peeled with heads removed

Freshly chopped parsley and 1 lemon, cut into 4 wedges, to garnish

Serves 4

BAKED SEAFOOD

Defrost 225 g cooked seafood cocktail and use this instead of the prawns. Add a handful of freshly chopped chives with the parsley.

MONKFISH KEBABS WITH LEMON & THYME

Monkfish has a fine flavour, and is ideal for kebabs as it keeps its nice, firm texture. If it's not available, use cod, haddock or another firm fish. Serve with warm crusty bread and a crisp green salad.

1 Preheat the grill to medium, and line the grill pan with kitchen foil.

2 Cut the fish fillets into chunks and place them in a bowl. Stir in the olive oil, garlic, lemon zest and juice, thyme, coriander and seasoning.

3 Thread the fish pieces onto 4 skewers. Secure the ends with lime wedges.

4 Grill, turning occasionally, for about 5–8 minutes. It is important to make sure that the fish does not over-cook.

650 g monkfish fillet

1 tablespoon olive oil

2 cloves garlic, crushed

Zest and juice of 1 lemon

2 tablespoons freshly chopped thyme

2 tablespoons freshly chopped coriander leaves

Salt and pepper, to taste

2 limes, quartered

Serves 4

HONEY-GLAZED CHICKEN WINGS

12 chicken wings

2½ cm piece root ginger, crushed

2 cloves garlic, crushed

1 teaspoon red chilli powder

2 teaspoons runny honey

2 teaspoons coarse grain mustard

1 teaspoon cider vinegar

2 tablespoons white wine vinegar

Salt and pepper, to taste

Serves 4

Chicken wings make a deliciously different starter, and this recipe transforms them into irresistibly tasty morsels. They're not for formal occasions – just eat them with your fingers.

1 Preheat the grill to medium. Line a large flameproof dish with kitchen foil.

2 Put the chicken wings into a bowl, add the remaining ingredients, and mix together thoroughly.

3 Arrange the coated wings in the dish, making sure that they don't overlap.

4 Cook under the grill for about 20 minutes, turning once or twice during cooking. Serve the wings hot or cold.

SAUTÉED CHICKEN LIVER WITH FENNEL

2 teaspoons corn oil

1 medium fennel, sliced

Salt and pepper

1 teaspoon plain flour

225 g chicken livers

3 tablespoons chopped parsley

1 tablespoon red wine vinegar

Serves 4

Chicken livers have a delicate taste compared to other offal. Liver is an excellent source of iron, vitamin B12 and protein, but make sure you don't overcook it as it can then become tough. The fennel adds a mild aniseed flavour to the dish.

1 Heat the oil over a moderately high heat. Stir-fry the fennel for about 3 minutes.

2 Add the salt and pepper to the flour and use this mixture to coat the liver.

3 Add the liver to the pan and cook it very quickly for about 5–10 minutes, stirring gently from time to time.

4 Slowly mix in the parsley and remove from heat. Pour in the vinegar. This should make a sizzling sound. Serve immediately.

Mini Kebabs with Yogurt Dip

These moist, beautifully flavoured lamb kebabs make a great start to a meal. The yogurt dip is a traditional accompaniment, and makes a cool, fresh contrast to the rich flavour of the meat. You could also serve this as a light lunch with pitta bread and mixed salad.

1 Preheat the grill to medium. Mix all the kebab ingredients together. As an alternative to lamb, you could use skinless minced chicken or turkey.

2 With your fingertips, shape a level tablespoon of the meat mixture around each skewer, forming a sausage shape.

3 Grill the kebabs for 10–15 minutes until they are well browned – turn them frequently to make sure they cook through.

4 Meanwhile, make the dip by mixing all the ingredients together, and chill in the refrigerator until the kebabs are ready to serve.

FOR THE KEBABS

300 g lean minced lamb

1 clove garlic, crushed

2½ cm piece of root ginger, crushed

½ teaspoon salt

2 teaspoons paprika

FOR THE DIP

2 tablespoons chopped fresh mint

2 tablespoons chopped flat-leaf parsley

1 teaspoon cumin seeds

150 ml low-fat natural yogurt

Serves 4

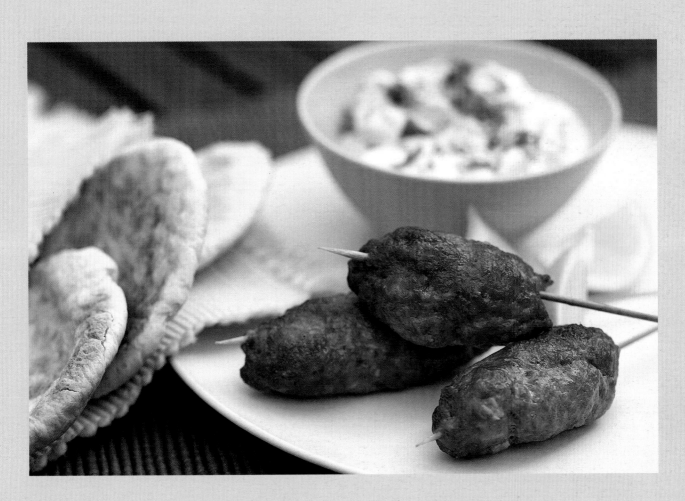

Falafels with Mint Dip

These crisp little savoury balls originate from the Middle East, and make an unusual starter. These are baked rather than fried, so they are much lower in fat than the traditional version.

FOR THE FALAFELS

1 teaspoon coriander seeds

½ teaspoon cumin seeds

2 teaspoons olive oil

1 small onion, finely chopped

1 garlic clove, crushed

410 g canned chickpeas

Large handful flat-leaf parsley, chopped

2 teaspoons self-raising flour

Large pinch of salt

FOR THE DIP

1 teaspoon mint sauce

150 g low-fat natural yogurt

Makes 12 falafels

1 Preheat the oven to 230°C, gas mark 8. Put the coriander and cumin seeds in a small, dry, frying pan and heat gently for 2–3 minutes until they become slightly brown and give off a fragrant smell.

2 Grind the seeds to a powder in a mortar and pestle or coffee grinder.

3 Heat the olive oil in the frying pan and fry the the onion and garlic for about 1–2 minutes, until they are softened.

4 In a bowl, mash the chickpeas to a pulp with a fork, leaving a few rougher pieces for texture. Add the ground roasted spices, onion and garlic mixture, chopped parsley, flour and salt.

5 Mix together well with your hands, and roll it into 12 small balls. Put these in an ovenproof dish and bake for 20 minutes.

6 Meanwhile, make the dipping sauce by mixing together the mint sauce and yogurt. Serve the falafels warm with the mint dip.

Roasted Baby Tomatoes & Aubergines

Oozing with aromatic juices, these roasted vegetables are flavoured with balsamic vinegar and make a colourful starter –they are best served with warm ciabatta bread.

4 baby aubergines, stalks removed

8 baby plum tomatoes, pierced once

2 tablespoons balsamic vinegar

Salt and pepper, to taste

Serves 4

1 Preheat the oven to 190°C, gas mark 5. Cut the baby aubergines into quarters lengthways.

2 Put them into an open ovenproof dish with the tomatoes and drizzle them with the balsamic vinegar. Season, then roast in the oven for 1 hour.

ROASTED FENNEL & AUBERGINES
Cut 2 fennel bulbs into quarters and 2 aubergines into bite-sized chunks. Lightly grease an oven-proof dish, season well and bake the vegetables in the oven (190°C, gas mark 5) for 30–40 minutes.

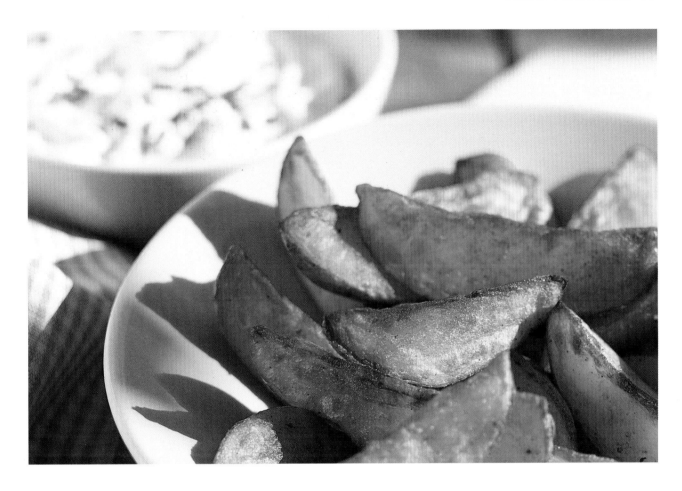

CRISPY POTATO WEDGES WITH CREAM & CHIVE DIP

These crunchy golden potato wedges are cleverly cooked so that they are healthily low in fat.

1 Preheat the grill to high and line the grill pan with kitchen foil.

2 Cut each potato lengthways into 8 wedges. Boil in lightly salted boiling water for 8-10 minutes or until they are just cooked. Drain.

3 Lightly grease the foil, and put the cooked potatoes into the grill pan. Season with the chilli powder and salt and pepper to taste.

4 Drizzle or brush the oil over the potato wedges, place under a hot grill and brown for 5–10 minutes.

5 Meanwhile, make the dip by mixing all the ingredients together. Serve the cooked wedges hot with the dip.

FOR THE POTATOES

3 baking potatoes, washed and scrubbed

2 tablespoons rapeseed or olive oil

½ teaspoon chilli powder

Salt and pepper, to taste

FOR THE DIP

55 g half-fat crème fraîche

175 g Greek yogurt

15 g snipped chives

Serves 4

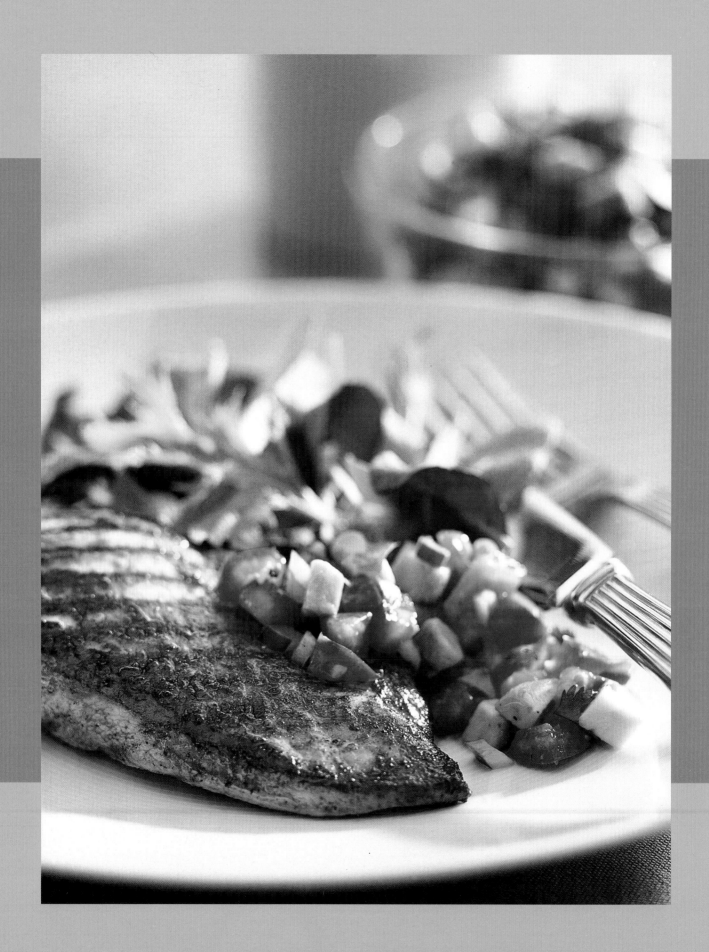

4 Main Meals

FISH

CHICKEN & POULTRY

MEAT

VEGETARIAN

TIGER PRAWN RISOTTO

Spray of pure vegetable oil

1 small onion, peeled and finely chopped

4 baby leeks, trimmed and finely sliced

250 g risotto rice, such as Arborio

900 ml hot stock made from 300 ml each
of fish stock, chicken stock and water

400 g raw tiger prawns, peeled

115 g frozen petit pois

40 g freshly grated Parmesan cheese

Serves 4

This fragrant risotto has a perfect texture – moist and creamy, with a satisfying 'bite' to the rice. If you prefer, you can use cooked prawns instead of raw – simply heat them through in the rice before serving.

1   Spray a large, heavy-based saucepan with a light coating of oil. Add the onion and leeks and cook over medium heat, until they are soft and translucent but not browned.

2   Add the rice and cook for 3 minutes stirring continuously, so that the grains are completely coated and slightly translucent.

3   Pour a ladleful of hot stock over the rice, stir and increase the heat so that the risotto bubbles gently. Stir continuously until the first batch of stock is absorbed. Continue adding and stirring in the stock, a ladleful at a time, until the rice is almost tender, but still *al dente*, or firm to the bite. Risotto should have a moist consistency, so, if necessary, add a little more stock.

4   Add the prawns and petit pois and stir into the rice. Turn up the heat and cook for a further 5 minutes until the prawns have cooked to a bright pink.

5   Remove from the heat, stir in the Parmesan cheese and serve immediately.

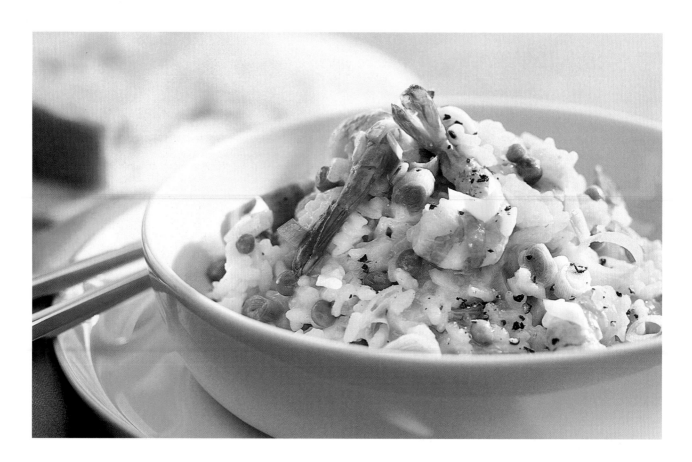

STIR-FRIED SQUID WITH LEMON GRASS & GINGER

Stir-fries are quick, healthy, and hold the crisp texture of their fresh vegetable ingredients. Here, lemon grass and ginger add a sharp burst of flavour to succulent baby squid. If you can't get pak choi, use spring greens or Chinese leaves instead.

1 Preheat a wok, then add the sesame oil. Heat the oil until it starts to smoke.

2 Stir in the lemon grass and ginger, quickly followed by the red pepper and spring onions.

3 Stir-fry for 1 minute, then add the squid rings, soy sauce and fish sauce, stirring continuously.

4 Cook for 4 minutes, toss in the pak choi and let it wilt slightly in the pan for a further minute. Add the egg noodles and mix well before serving.

1 tablespoon toasted sesame oil

2 stalks of lemon grass, outer leaves removed, finely chopped, then crushed with the blade of a knife

5 cm piece of fresh ginger root, peeled then finely chopped

2 small red peppers, deseeded and diced

12 spring onions, chopped

450 g baby squid, sliced into 1 cm rings

2 teaspoons soy sauce

½ teaspoon fish sauce (nam pla)

315 g pak choi, stalks and leaves trimmed and roughly chopped

225 g medium egg noodles, cooked according to the packet instructions

Serves 4

SMOKED FISH PARCELS

Smoked cod topped with a crunchy oatmeal crust and baked in a foil parcel makes a fragrant treat – especially if you use naturally smoked fillets, which have a more subtle, delicate flavour than those dyed with artificial colour. Serve with steamed new potatoes and baby carrots.

1 Preheat the oven to 190°C, gas mark 5.

2 Cut a 45 cm x 45 cm piece of kitchen foil, and spread it out flat. Place the spring onions, button mushrooms and tarragon in the centre, then add the pieces of smoked cod. Season with black pepper.

3 Mix the medium and rough oatmeals together and press the mixture onto the flesh of the fish fillets to make a crust.

4 Turn the edges of the foil up, and pour the wine around the base of the fish. Seal the parcel with a double fold on the top and ends, leaving enough space for steam to expand.

5 Bake in the oven for half an hour, remove the tarragon and serve the fish on a bed of the baked onions and mushrooms.

6 spring onions, chopped

175 g button mushrooms, sliced

Sprig of fresh tarragon

600 g smoked cod fillet, skinned and cut into 4 pieces

Black pepper, to taste

25 g medium-ground oatmeal

15 g rough-cut oatmeal

50 ml dry white wine

Serves 4

PAN-FRIED COD WITH PESTO

2 tablespoons olive oil

Salt and pepper, to taste

800 g cod fillet, skinned and cut into 4 pieces

Juice of one fresh lime

FOR THE PESTO

60 ml olive oil

4 x 15 g packs fresh basil leaves

2 cloves garlic, peeled

80 g pine nuts or peanuts

30 g Parmesan cheese

50 ml cold water

Black pepper, to taste

Serves 4

Savour the aromatic scents, flavours and colours of Mediterranean cooking in this quickly prepared dish, and serve it with a fresh tomato salad and ciabatta bread. The pesto sauce is a low-fat version of the regional classic, and tastes just as good.

1 Heat a large, non-stick frying pan and add the olive oil. Season the cod fillets and pour half the lime juice over them. Pan-fry over a medium heat, skin side down, and leave to cook for about 5 minutes.

2 Meanwhile, put the ingredients for the pesto into a blender and process until they are combined, but still retain a crumbly texture.

3 Turn the fillets and pour the remaining lime juice over them. Fry for another 4–5 minutes, until the fish is just cooked. Add a little cold water if the fish begins to stick to the pan.

4 Slide the cooked fillets gently onto a warmed serving dish, skin side down, and coat them with the pesto sauce. Serve immediately.

BALSAMIC SALMON STEAKS

4 salmon steaks, each about 175 g

FOR THE MARINADE

2 tablespoons balsamic vinegar

2 tablespoons soy sauce

1 tablespoon olive oil

2 teaspoons coarse grain mustard

2 garlic cloves, peeled and crushed

2 tablespoons fresh dill, finely chopped

Salt and pepper, to taste

Serves 4

Salmon is justly prized for its sweetly succulent flesh, and this imaginative recipe adds an intense, complex range of extra flavours. You can either soak the fish steaks in the rich, aromatic marinade, or cover them with the mixture and grill straight away. Either way, they taste wonderful.

1 Place the salmon steaks in a non-metallic dish. In a separate bowl, mix together the vinegar, soy sauce, oil, mustard, garlic, dill and seasoning.

2 Pour the mixture over the salmon, turning it over to coat both sides. If marinating, cover the salmon and refrigerate for 30 minutes.

3 Preheat the grill, and line the grill tray with kitchen foil. Lift the salmon out of the marinade and place on the grill tray.

4 Grill under a moderate heat for about 4–5 minutes each side, turning once.

Grilled Halibut with Red Pepper Sauce

If you're planning a special meal, try these tender cutlets of halibut garnished with a sizzling, spicy-sweet pepper sauce. Serve with wild rice, if available, and steamed green vegetables.

1 Preheat the grill. Place the peppers skin side up on the grill tray, and cook under a high heat for about 15 minutes, or until the skins are blackened. Put them inside a plastic bag, and leave to cool for 10 minutes.

2 Meanwhile, line the grill tray with kitchen foil. Brush the cutlets lightly on both sides with the olive oil, and spread the garlic and ginger over them. Season and put them on the grill tray. Grill for 5–6 minutes on each side, turning once, until the flesh flakes easily.

3 Heat the oil in a frying pan and sauté the onions for about 2–3 minutes until they are translucent. Add the curry paste and cook for 1 minute.

4 Peel the peppers and put them in a food processor with the onion mixture, herbs, and lime juice. Blend until smooth and add seasoning if necessary.

5 Serve the fish with the red pepper sauce, garnished with lime wedges.

4 halibut cutlets, about 175 g each

1 tablespoon olive oil

1 clove garlic, peeled and crushed

1 teaspoon crushed ginger

Salt and pepper, to taste

FOR THE PEPPER SAUCE

2 teaspoons olive oil

1 small onion, chopped

1 teaspoon Thai red curry paste

3 red peppers, halved and deseeded

Fresh basil leaves, torn

Sprig of fresh thyme or a pinch of dried thyme

2 tablespoons lime juice

Lime wedges, to garnish

Serves 4

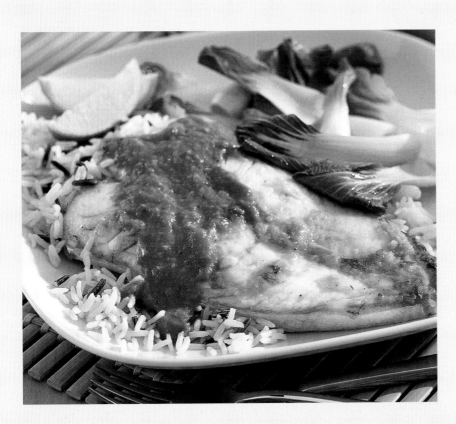

FETTUCCINE WITH SALMON, ASPARAGUS & LEMON

450 g fresh salmon fillets

350 g fresh fettuccine

10 fresh asparagus tips, cut in half

Juice of 2 large lemons (or 3 small)

150 ml half-fat crème fraîche

150 ml low-fat fromage frais

Black pepper to taste

Fresh rocket leaves, to garnish

Serves 4

Pasta and salmon are perfect partners and this light, fragrant dish proves the point. Freshly cooked fettucine is coated in a creamy, but healthily low-fat, sauce which is studded with luscious asparagus tips and flakes of fresh, briny salmon. All you need to serve it with is a simple salad of mixed leaves.

1 Preheat the oven to 190°C, gas mark 5. Wrap the salmon in kitchen foil and bake for 30 minutes. Leave to cool for 10 minutes, remove any skin, and roughly flake the flesh. Set aside. Instead of using fresh salmon fillets, you can also use 125 g of smoked salmon pieces – they're much cheaper and a really good buy.

2 Meanwhile bring a large pan of lightly salted water to the boil, and cook the fettucine for 2–3 minutes until *al dente*. Drain and set aside.

3 Simmer the asparagus tips gently for 5 minutes, then drain.

4 In a large saucepan, combine the lemon juice, crème fraîche and fromage frais and cook over a low heat for 1–2 minutes.

5 Add the fettuccine then fold in the asparagus tips and salmon flakes. Mix thoroughly and season with black pepper. If using smoked salmon pieces, heat through for 1 minute before serving.

6 Serve immediately, garnished with fresh rocket leaves.

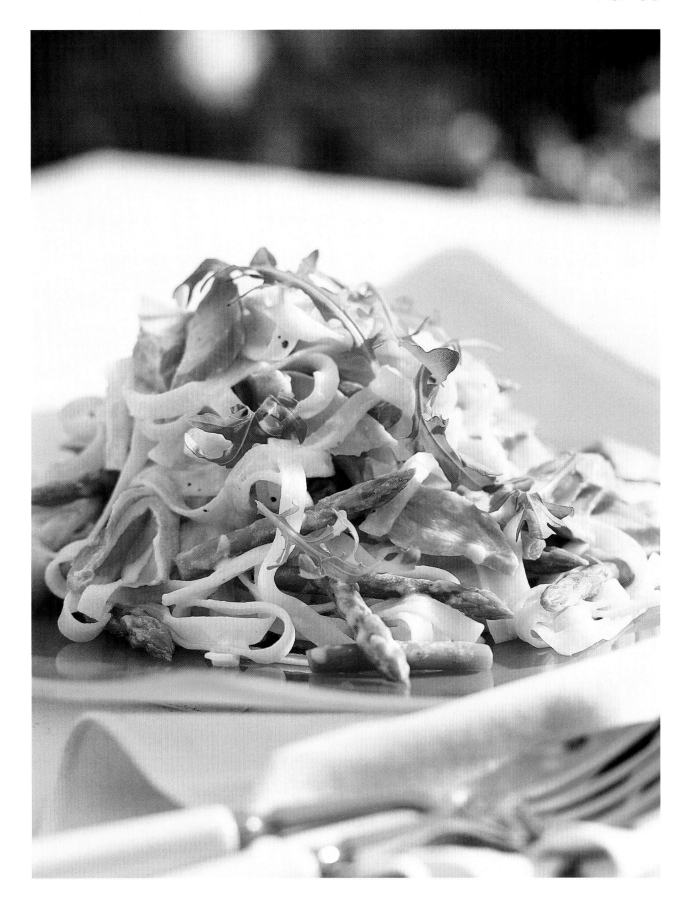

CORIANDER CHICKEN WITH ORANGE

55 g dried currants

200 ml unsweetened orange juice

1 tablespoon olive oil

4 large chicken thighs, skinned

1 large red onion, sliced into large petals

4 whole garlic cloves, peeled

1 teaspoon coriander seeds, freshly crushed

2 medium red chillies, deseeded and finely chopped

2 cinnamon sticks

55 g whole blanched almonds

2 large oranges, peeled and white pith removed, roughly chopped

300 ml chicken stock

Sprigs of fresh mint, tied

Serves 4

Plump chicken thighs are scented with a medley of spices and citrus flavours. As the garlic cloves are cooked whole, they are not very pungent, and are meltingly soft and juicy to eat. The chicken is cooked on the bone, and makes a beautifully rich sauce that requires no extra thickening. Serve on a bed of rice or steamed couscous.

1 Soak the currants overnight in half the orange juice, or for at least 1 hour.

2 Preheat the oven to 200°C, gas mark 6. Heat the olive oil in a shallow, non-stick casserole dish and sauté the chicken for 2 minutes. Add the onions, garlic and coriander. Cook until the onions are soft and starting to brown.

3 Add the chillies, cinnamon sticks, almonds, currants, the remaining orange juice, chopped oranges, chicken stock and mint.

4 Bring to the boil, then transfer the casserole to the oven. Cook uncovered for 40 minutes. Discard the mint and cinnamon sticks and serve.

CHICKEN BREASTS WITH SALSA

2 X 150 g skinned and boned chicken breasts

1 tablespoon corn or rapeseed oil

FOR THE MARINADE

Juice of 1 lime

1 teaspoon tomato purée

1 tablespoon Worcestershire sauce

½ teaspoon cayenne pepper

The tangy salsa topping makes a splash of colour on these tender chicken breasts and enhances the flavours of the peppery marinade. This is a relaxed, informal dish, ideal for eating outdoors. Serve it with rice and mixed vegetables, a mixed bean salad, tucked into pockets of warmed pitta bread or folded inside tortilla wraps.

1 Combine the marinade ingredients in an ovenproof dish and mix in the chicken breasts so they are completely coated. Refrigerate overnight, if possible, otherwise marinate for at least 1 hour.

2 Make the salsa. To loosen the skin from the tomatoes, make a small incision in the skin of each one, then plunge them into boiling water for 1 minute. Lift them out with a slotted spoon, and immediately plunge them into cold water. Leave them in the cold water for about 1 minute, then lift them out. Remove the skin from the tomatoes, chop the flesh finely and transfer to a bowl.

3 Add the remaining salsa ingredients and mix together thoroughly. Cover and leave aside to allow the flavours to develop.

4 Brush the surface of a non-stick griddle pan with the oil and place over high heat until it is very hot. Add the chicken breasts and lower the heat to medium. Griddle for 5–6 minutes on both sides until they are fully cooked and slightly charred. Serve hot with the salsa.

BARBECUED CHICKEN KEBABS

If you prefer, you can barbecue the chicken. Cut the breasts into cubes before marinating, then thread them onto skewers, adding alternating pieces of vegetables such as mushroom, onions and peppers. Baste with the remaining marinade, and cook until the juices run clear when pierced with a knife.

FOR THE SALSA

2–3 large tomatoes

1 large, ripe avocado, flesh removed and cut into small dice

1 small red onion, finely diced

40 g fresh coriander leaves, chopped

Juice of 1 lime

Dash of hot pepper sauce, to taste

Salt and pepper, to taste

Serves 2

CHICKEN WITH GINGER

The luscious flavours of aromatic ginger combined with sweet honey and tangy lemons make this dish elegant enough for a dinner party. But it is also an inexpensive choice for a relaxed family occasion. Though honey is used here, it is less likely to make your blood sugar rise quickly when cooked with other ingredients.

1 Combine the ingredients for the marinade in a non-metallic dish that will hold the chicken comfortably. Using a sharp knife, make several deep cuts in the upper sides of the chicken breasts. Place them in the marinade, cut side down. Leave overnight, or for at least 4 hours, turning occasionally.

2 Preheat the oven to 190°C, gas mark 5. Cut four 30 cm x 30 cm square pieces of kitchen foil, and brush with the sunflower oil.

3 Remove the chicken breasts from the marinade and wrap each one loosely in foil. Place the foil parcels on a non-stick baking tray.

4 Roast the chicken breasts in the centre of the oven for 25 minutes or until they are cooked through (the juices should run clear when the chicken is pierced with a knife).

5 While the chicken is cooking, pour the remaining marinade into a small pan, add the cornflour paste, and cook gently, stirring all the time, until the mixture boils and thickens. Season with salt and pepper to taste.

6 Unwrap the foil parcels and serve the chicken with the sauce poured over, and garnished with the lemon zest.

FOR THE MARINADE

150 ml freshly squeezed lemon juice

25 g preserved ginger, finely chopped

25 g clear honey

2 cloves garlic, peeled and crushed

2 tablespoons dark soy sauce

FOR THE CHICKEN

4 x 175 g skinned and boned chicken breasts

1 tablespoon sunflower oil

15 g cornflour, mixed to a thin paste with a little water

Salt and pepper, to taste

2 teaspoons finely grated lemon zest, to garnish

Serves 4

CHICKEN WITH CARDAMOM

300 g skinned and boned chicken breasts, chopped into bite-size pieces

Spray of pure vegetable oil

8 whole black cardamom pods

3 cm stick cinnamon

1 bay leaf

4 whole cloves

2 small onions, finely chopped

55 g ground almonds

3 cloves garlic, peeled and crushed

2½ cm piece of fresh ginger, peeled and coarsely grated

1 teaspoon ground cumin

280 g low-fat natural yogurt

200 ml chicken stock

85 g raisins

20 g roasted whole almonds, crushed

Serves 4

Succulent pieces of chicken breasts are scented with a heady mix of fragrant spices. Serve with basmati rice cooked with a pinch of golden saffron, and a green vegetable such as steamed French beans. Black cardamom pods are widely available in Asian food stores, as well as supermarkets (green cardamom pods do not make a suitable substitute).

1 Choose a large, shallow, non-stick pan with a close-fitting lid, and spray the base with pure vegetable oil. Heat gently, then add the chicken pieces.

2 Cook over a low heat until the chicken starts to colour, stir in the whole spices and onions, and cook for 3–4 minutes.

3 Add the ground almonds, garlic, ginger and cumin and cook for a further 3 minutes. Pour in the yogurt and chicken stock gradually, stirring continuously while doing so.

4 Cover, reduce the heat to low, and cook gently for 20 minutes. Add the raisins, mix thoroughly, then cover and cook for another 10 minutes.

5 Remove the whole spices. Serve the chicken hot on a bed of rice, sprinkled with the crushed almonds.

TURKEY WITH RED ONION & WATERCRESS SALAD

FOR THE TURKEY

2 tablespoons plain flour

1 teaspoon paprika

1 teaspoon Cajun seasoning

1 teaspoon dried mixed herbs

Salt and pepper, to taste

4 X 170 g skinned turkey breasts, cut into 1 cm wide strips

2 tablespoons corn or rapeseed oil

Turkey breast has a more intense flavour than chicken, but is just as healthily low in fat. Ready-skinned and boned breasts are available in convenient packs all year round at most supermarkets, and they are perfect for this tasty, char-grilled dish.

1 Mix the flour with the paprika, Cajun seasoning, herbs, and salt and pepper to taste. Use the mixture to coat the strips of turkey breast.

2 Pour the oil into a heavy-based non-stick frying pan, and place over high heat. Add the turkey strips, and lower the heat to medium.

3 Fry the turkey strips in the oil for 3–4 minutes, until they are crisp and golden.

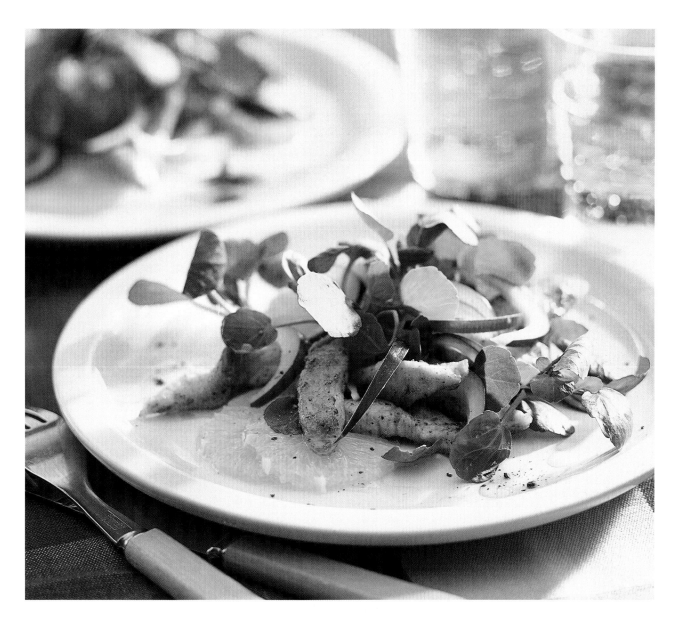

4 Meanwhile, make the salad. Mix together the watercress, red onion, lime juice and black pepper.

5 To serve, divide the turkey between 4 warmed dinner plates. Arrange the orange slices on the side, and scatter the watercress salad on top.

FOR THE SALAD

80 g packet fresh watercress

1 large red onion, sliced

Juice of 2 fresh limes

Black pepper, to taste

2 oranges, peeled and sliced into rounds, to serve

Serves 4

TURKEY FRICASÉE WITH OLIVE OIL MASH

FOR THE FRICASÉE

1 tablespoon plain flour

Salt and pepper

2 tablespoons corn or rapeseed oil

1 medium onion, finely chopped

2 cloves garlic, crushed

1 chicken stock cube

4 skinless turkey breasts (weighing around 170g each), cut into bite-sized chunks

3 medium carrots, diced

1 green pepper, diced

110 g Greek yogurt

4 tablespoons fresh parsley, chopped

FOR THE MASH

450 g potatoes, peeled and chopped

½ teaspoon garlic salt, or to taste

150 ml skimmed milk

1 tablespoon low fat soft cheese

1 teaspoon mixed dried herbs

2 tablespoon extra virgin olive oil

Few sprigs fresh parsley

Serves 4

The definition of a fricasée is a white stew of poultry and vegetables which are first fried in butter and then cooked in stock with the addition of cream and egg yolks. This recipe is adapted to keep the saturated fat down by using Greek yogurt and chicken stock to make an appetising sauce for turkey, carrots and green peppers. It goes extremely well with this soft Mediterranean mashed potato.

1 Mix the flour with the seasoning and use this to coat the turkey pieces.

2 Heat the oil in a non-stick pan. Add the onion and garlic and fry for a few minutes to soften them.

3 Make the chicken stock cube up to 250 ml with hot water.

4 Add the turkey to the pan and brown over a medium heat, adding a little of the stock if it sticks to the bottom.

5 Stir in the carrots and remaining stock. Cover and simmer for 5 minutes.

6 Meanwhile, boil the potatoes with the garlic salt until tender.

7 Add the peppers to the fricasée and allow to cook, covered, for a further 5 minutes.

8 Stir in the Greek yogurt and fresh parsley. Warm through and adjust the seasoning if necessary.

9 Drain and mash the potatoes with the milk, cheese, herbs and olive oil. Serve hot with the fricasée and garnish with fresh parsley sprigs.

COD FRICASÉE

Use 4 medium fillets of cod instead of the turkey and cut them into bite sized chunks. Coat them in the seasoned flour as above and fry with the onion and garlic until just cooked. Remove the fish and follow the method above until the fricasée is cooked through. Add the cooked fish to the yogurt and serve with the mash.

DUCK BREASTS WITH COCONUT

Flavoured with spicy-sweet Thai curry paste and reduced-fat coconut milk (both available from large supermarkets and Asian food stores), these duck breasts are succulent and fragrant; serve them simply on a bed of steamed basmati rice. By removing the skin and surface fat, you reduce the fat content considerably.

1 Preheat the grill to high, then place the duck slices on the grill tray, and cook for about 4 minutes.

2 Warm the coconut milk in a wok or large, heavy-based frying pan, then add the curry paste and the mangetout. Simmer for one minute.

3 Stir in the duck, tomatoes and basil leaves, and simmer for 10 minutes more until the meat absorbs the flavours. Serve immediately.

300 g duck breasts, skin and surface fat removed, cut into 1 cm thick slices

300 ml reduced-fat coconut milk

2 teaspoons red Thai curry paste

150 g mangetout

12 cherry tomatoes, halved

Handful of fresh basil leaves

Serves 4

SWEET & SOUR DUCK

You can use fresh or canned pineapple in this easy version of a classic sweet and sour dish – both give excellent results. Serve with plain steamed rice or egg noodles.

1 Preheat the grill to medium hot, and place the duck breasts on the grill tray. Cook for about 5–6 minutes each side, depending on their thickness.

2 In a large saucepan, heat the sesame oil, then add the diced peppers and cook until they are softened.

3 Drain the juice from the pineapple and add the juice to the peppers. Mix in the wine vinegar, brown sugar, tomato purée, soy sauce, and sherry, then stir in the cornflour paste. Continue stirring until the sauce turns clear.

4 Add the pineapple pieces to the sauce, and cook for 3 minutes. Mix in the grated carrot, and cook for a further 2 minutes before serving.

5 Spoon the sweet and sour sauce onto a serving plate, and arrange the slices of duck breast over the top. Sprinkle with sesame seeds to garnish.

4 x 115 g duck breasts, skin and surface fat removed

FOR THE SWEET AND SOUR SAUCE

1 teaspoon sesame oil

2 bell peppers (one red, one yellow), deseeded and finely diced

400 g fresh pineapple, diced and soaked in 150 ml unsweetened pineapple juice (or 450 g can pineapple chunks)

4 tablespoons white wine vinegar

15 g brown sugar

1 tablespoon tomato purée

3 tablespoons soy sauce

2 tablespoons dry sherry

55 g cornflour mixed to a thin paste with 75 ml water

1 large carrot, grated

10 g sesame seeds, to garnish

Serves 4

SMOKED SAUSAGE CASSOULET

Traditionally a rustic French dish, this easy version makes a warming family meal on cold winter evenings. It's packed with good flavours, and you'll need chunks of soda bread or crusty French bread to soak up the juices. If you can't get shallots, use 3 small onions, peeled and cut into quarters. Accompany the cassoulet with lightly steamed cauliflower and broccoli florets.

Spray of pure vegetable oil

1 garlic clove, peeled and crushed

12 whole shallots, peeled

250 g fresh, low-fat spicy or garlic-flavoured sausages, cut into chunks

85 g dried sausage such as Chorizo or Kabanos, cut into pieces

400 g can butter beans, drained

400 g can flageolet beans, drained

2 x 400 g cans tomatoes

Pinch of mixed herbs

1 tablespoon tomato purée

1 tablespoon Dijon mustard

Salt and pepper to taste

2 tablespoons chopped parsley, to garnish

Serves 4–6

1 Coat the base of a large saucepan with a spray of pure vegetable oil. Cook the garlic and shallots (or onions if using) for 2–3 minutes over a medium heat, until they are softened but not browned.

2 Add the fresh and dried sausage pieces and mix thoroughly. Cook for 5 minutes until the sausage is lightly coloured, then add the beans, tomatoes, herbs, purée, mustard and seasoning.

3 Bring the mixture to the boil, then reduce the heat. Cover and simmer gently for 20 minutes to allow the flavours to develop.

4 Sprinkle with the chopped parsley and serve immediately.

ITALIAN MEATBALLS

Meatballs are a universal family favourite, originating from the south of Italy, and full of the sunny flavours typical of that region. These are made with healthily lean pork and are served with penne, but any pasta is suitable.

FOR THE MEATBALLS

400 g lean minced pork

25 g fresh breadcrumbs

1 egg white

3 teaspoons pesto sauce

Salt and pepper, to taste

FOR THE TOMATO SAUCE

1 small onion, finely chopped

1 clove garlic, crushed

450 ml passata

50 ml wine (red or white)

350 g penne, cooked *al dente*, to serve

Serves 4

1 Preheat the oven to 190°C, gas mark 5. In a large bowl, combine all the ingredients for the meatballs and mix them thoroughly with your hands.

2 Place the mixture on a square of greaseproof paper, and pat it out into a 2 cm thick square. Cut it out into 2 cm cubes, then, with wet hands, roll each cube into a firmly packed ball. This way, you'll get evenly sized meatballs.

3 Place the meatballs in a greased ovenproof dish and bake for 20 minutes.

4 Put the ingredients for the tomato sauce in a pan, and bring to the boil. Lower the heat, and simmer, uncovered, until the meatballs are ready.

5 Transfer the meatballs into the pan of tomato sauce and simmer for a further 10 minutes. Serve with the pasta.

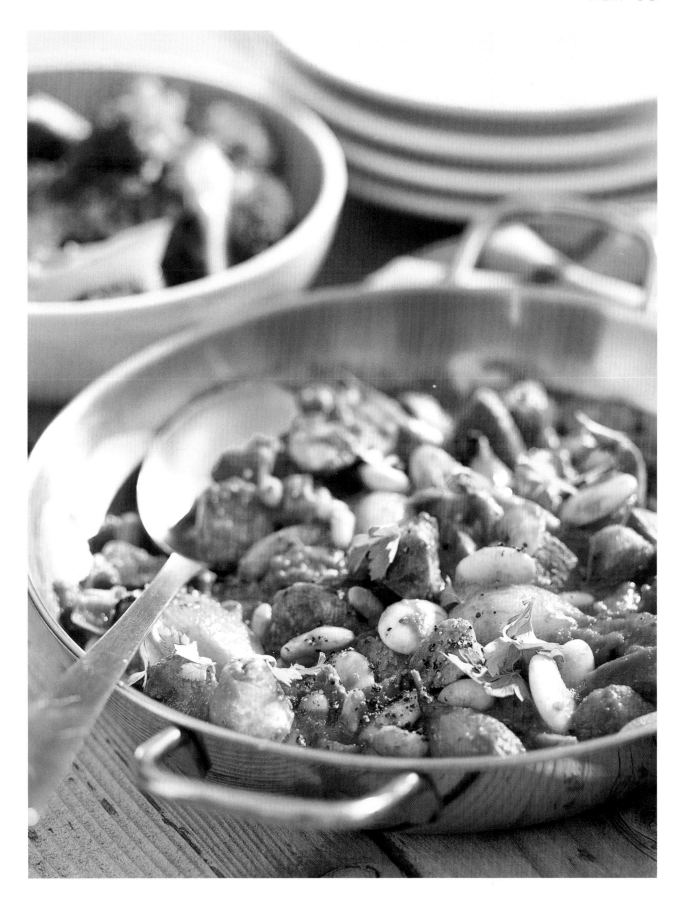

BEEF WITH GREEN PEPPER & NOODLES

450 g rump steak, cut into thin strips

3 tablespoons soy sauce

1 tablespoon dry sherry

2 tablespoons vegetable oil

1 leek, thinly sliced into rings

1 green pepper, cut into chunks

2½ cm piece root ginger, peeled and sliced into thin strips

75 g bean sprouts

2 large tomatoes, cut into wedges

2 teaspoons sesame oil

350 g noodles

Salt and pepper

Serves 4

This tangy dish is delicious and cooks quickly once the meat is marinated, which can be done long beforehand. The beef is cut into thin strips so it takes very little time to cook. Noodles and other pasta have a low glycaemic index and if you use rice noodles, you'll be going for an even lower fat option.

1 Coat the meat well with the mixture of the soy sauce and the sherry. Leave to marinate for 30 minutes. Drain the beef, reserving the marinade.

2 Cook the noodles in a large saucepan of boiling water, following the instructions on the packet. Drain and set aside.

3 Heat the oil in a wok and stir fry the meat for 2–3 minutes on high. Remove with a slotted spoon and keep warm.

4 Add the leeks, pepper and ginger and stir-fry for 4 minutes. Next add the marinade, cooked beef and the bean sprouts. Cook for 2–3 minutes until the vegetables are cooked but crisp.

5 Heat the sesame oil in a wok or large pan. Stir in the noodles, season and serve with the beef.

GRIDDLED FILLET STEAK WITH FIELD MUSHROOMS

450 g fillet steak

30 g unsalted butter

1 medium onion, finely chopped

450 g field mushrooms, sliced

1 tablespoon tomato purée

1 tablespoon French mustard

2 tablespoons plain flour, or as required

50 ml half-fat crème fraîche

Salt and pepper

Serves 4

A tantalising mix of wild mushrooms with fillet steak, all coated in a rich creamy sauce. Serve this with a pile of fresh vegetables such as broccoli or mangetout and balance it with some new boiled potatoes in their skins.

1 Wipe and trim the steak. Beat it flat and cut into bite-sized pieces.

2 Heat half the butter and fry the onions and mushrooms over a low heat until just beginning to colour.

3 Stir in the tomato purée, mustard and enough flour to absorb the fat. Continue frying over a low heat for a couple of minutes, then carefully blend in the crème fraîche. Remove from heat.

4 Heat the remaining butter in a clean non-stick pan and fry the meat over a high heat till brown. Add a little water if it sticks to the bottom.

5 Blend the beef into the sauce, season and serve.

LAMB WITH APRICOTS

Tender lamb and succulent apricots complement each other beautifully in this recipe, and produce a wonderfully rich, aromatic sauce. You'll need to soak this up with saffron-flavoured rice, mashed potato or steamed couscous. Serve with some lightly steamed green beans or mangetout to give a fresh, green contrast.

1 Marinate the apricots, orange rind and raisins in the cider and orange juice for 1 hour (or overnight if you are using ordinary dried apricots).

2 Preheat the oven to 180°C, gas mark 4. Spray the base of a large casserole pan with a thin layer of oil, and brown the meat lightly.

3 Add the onion, mushrooms, pepper and garlic and cook for 5 minutes.

4 Add the stock, paprika, apricot mixture (including the marinade), bay leaves and Worcestershire Sauce.

5 Cover and cook in the oven for 1 hour. Remember to remove the bay leaves before serving.

115 g 'ready-to-eat' dried apricots

Grated rind and juice of 1 orange

25 g seedless raisins

400 ml dry cider

Spray of pure vegetable oil

400 g lamb fillet, trimmed and cut into 1cm thick slices

1 large onion, chopped

115 g button mushrooms

1 large yellow pepper, sliced

1 clove garlic, peeled and crushed

300 ml beef or lamb stock

Pinch of paprika

2 bay leaves

1 tablespoon Worcestershire Sauce

Serves 4

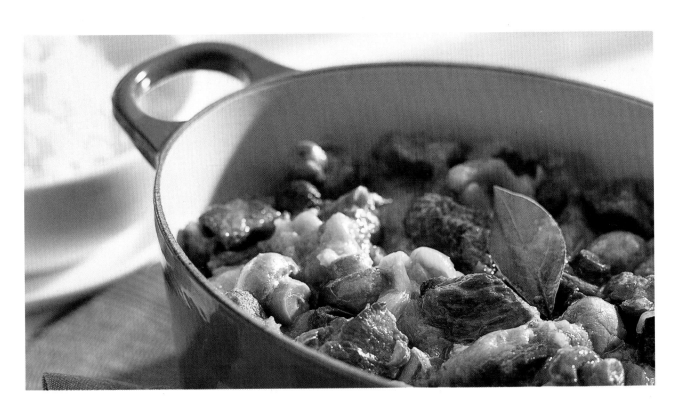

Lamb Baked in Yogurt

2¼ kg leg of lamb, fat and skin removed

FOR THE MARINADE

55 g ground almonds

2 large onions peeled and coarsely chopped

8 cloves garlic, peeled

10 cm root ginger, peeled and chopped

4 green chillies, deseeded and chopped

500 ml low-fat plain yogurt

2 tablespoons ground cumin

4 teaspoons ground coriander

½ teaspoon cayenne pepper

1 teaspoon salt

½ teaspoon garam masala

2 tablespoons plain yogurt sprinkled with a pinch ground cumin, to serve

Serves 6–8

Cook this delicious recipe for a special dinner party. Moist, succulent, leg of lamb is baked in a coating of creamy yogurt and aromatic spices. Vegetable Pilaf (see page 67) would be a perfect accompaniment.

1 Wipe the leg of lamb with a cloth and place it in a non-stick roasting pan.

2 Combine the ground almonds, onions, garlic, ginger and chillies with 3 tablespoons of the yogurt in a blender and liquidise to a smooth paste.

3 Put the remaining yogurt in a bowl, and stir in the paste mixture, ground cumin, coriander, cayenne pepper, salt and garam masala. Mix thoroughly.

4 With a small, sharp, knife, make deep slashes in the surface of the lamb, and push the yogurt mixture into the gashes. Spread the remaining mixture over the meat, ensuring it is all covered. Cover with cling film and refrigerate for 24 hours.

5 Preheat the oven to 200°C, gas mark 6. Remove the cling film and cover the dish tightly with kitchen foil or a lid. Bake, covered, for 1½ hours basting 2–3 times with the sauce. Uncover, and bake for a further 45 minutes. Remove from the oven and let the meat rest for 15 minutes in a warm place before serving with the yogurt and cumin.

Venison in Red Wine

1 tablespoon corn oil

600 g venison, fat removed, diced into 2 cm cubes

1 large onion, chopped

3 medium tomatoes, skins removed (see page 56) and chopped

1 bouquet garni

Small piece of cinnamon stick

5 pickled walnuts, sliced

125 ml red wine

200 ml strong beef stock

Serves 4

Farmed venison is now widely available from large supermarkets, and makes an excellent alternative to beef – it is healthy, low in fat, and has a superb flavour. Serve this fragrant casserole with Parsnip Croquettes (see page 78), creamy mashed potatoes and a lightly cooked green vegetable.

1 Preheat the oven to 180°C, gas mark 4. Heat a large, non-stick flameproof casserole dish, add the oil and stir in the diced venison. Sauté for 2–3 minutes to lightly brown the meat.

2 Add the onions, tomatoes, bouquet garni, cinnamon, walnuts, wine and stock and mix together thoroughly.

3 Bake in the oven for 1½ hours, and serve immediately.

BROCCOLI & HERB PASTA

Use a single, fresh green vegetable for this pasta dish, as this keeps the flavour clean and distinctive. Broccoli is used here, but you could use any vegetable you like, such as courgettes, cauliflower, green beans or broad beans. Like the pasta, the vegetable should be cooked al dente.

1 Cook the pasta shells in a large pan of boiling salted water for about 12 minutes or until just tender, and drain them well.

2 While the pasta is cooking, steam the broccoli until it is cooked, but still has a firm 'bite'. Meanwhile, heat the oil in a large non-stick pan and sauté the onion and garlic over a gentle heat for about 5 minutes or until soft.

4 Add the tomatoes, herbs, broccoli and seasoning and mix gently but thoroughly. Mix in the cooked pasta and reheat if necessary and serve with a sprinkling of fresh basil and Parmesan cheese.

300 g dried pasta shells

450 g broccoli florets

1 tablespoon rapeseed oil

1 medium onion, finely chopped

2 cloves garlic, peeled and crushed

400 g can chopped tomatoes

1 teaspoon Herbes de Provence

Salt and pepper, to taste

25 g freshly grated Parmesan cheese and a few chopped fresh basil leaves, to serve

Serves 4

VEGETABLE PILAF

The saffron in this recipe gives this dish a beautiful yellow colour, but if you prefer, you can use a pinch of turmeric instead.

1 Drain the rice and set aside.

2 In a large saucepan, heat the oil gently, and sprinkle in the cumin seeds, stirring continuously for a few seconds.

3 Add the sliced onion, peppercorns, cloves, cinnamon and bay leaf, mix well then stir in the vegetables, salt and soaked rice.

4 Add the vegetable stock and saffron, bring to the boil, then reduce the heat.

5 Cover tightly and cook over a low heat for about 15–20 minutes, until all the water has been absorbed.

225 g basmati rice, washed and soaked in water for 1 hour

1 teaspoon corn or sunflower oil

1 teaspoon cumin seeds

1 small onion, sliced

12 peppercorns

4 cloves

1 stick cinnamon

1 bay leaf

4 large carrots, finely diced

115 g frozen peas

115 g frozen baby broad beans

200 g broccoli florets

½ teaspoon salt

600 ml vegetable stock (or water)

Few saffron threads

Serves 4

POLENTA WITH TOMATOES, PORCINI & GOAT'S CHEESE

500 g ready-cooked polenta

50 g sun-dried tomatoes, non-oily

25 g porcini (dried mushrooms)

1 tablespoon olive or rapeseed oil

Salt and pepper, to taste

115 g goat's cheese, cut into cubes

4 sprigs fresh basil, to garnish

Serves 2

Nothing could be more deceptively simple than this polenta recipe, but it is utterly sophisticated. Use the ready-cooked polenta, which is now widely available vacuum-packed in large supermarkets. This makes a delicious lunch or supper dish.

1   Drop the pouch of polenta into a large pan of boiling water. Lower the heat and simmer gently for 30 minutes.

2   Meanwhile, soak the sun-dried tomatoes and the mushrooms in a little water for 30 minutes, according to the packet instructions. Drain and reserve the liquid.

3   Cut the pack of polenta open, and transfer the contents to a saucepan. Stir in the oil, tomatoes and mushrooms with 1 tablespoon of the reserved liquid. Season to taste.

4   Finally, stir in the diced goat's cheese and serve the polenta immediately, garnished with fresh basil.

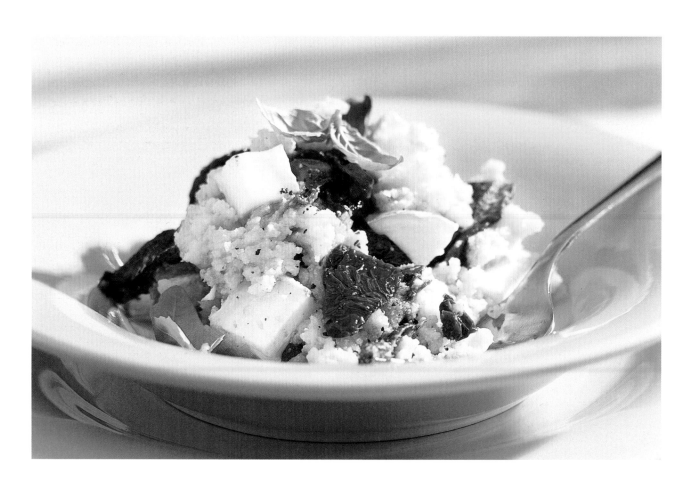

POLENTA BRUSCHETTAS WITH MEDITERRANEAN VEGETABLES

Made from maize or corn meal, polenta has a distinctive golden colour and is a favourite dish from Northern Italy. As the traditional method requires long cooking, use instant polenta — it's widely available in supermarkets. These delicious bruschettas are flavoured with Parmesan cheese, and topped with sunny Mediterranean vegetables.

1 Cook the polenta according to the packet instructions. Once it comes to the boil, stir vigorously with a wooden spoon for about 5 minutes.

2 Add the Parmesan cheese, season to taste, and turn into a shallow, lightly oiled dish and allow to set.

3 Meanwhile, cook the vegetables. Heat the oil in a medium-sized pan, add the onion and sauté gently for 2–3 minutes until softened but not browned.

4 Add the green pepper, courgettes and aubergines and sauté for a further 5 minutes. Add the tomatoes, herbs and seasoning. Bring to the boil, then lower the heat and simmer, uncovered, until the vegetables are tender, but not mushy.

5 To make the bruschettas, cut the set polenta into 4 wedges or 12 slices and brush them with a little olive oil. Grill or griddle until golden.

6 Serve covered with the vegetables, garnished with fresh basil leaves.

FOR THE BRUSCHETTAS

225 g instant polenta

25 g freshly grated Parmesan cheese

Salt and pepper, to taste

1 tablespoon extra virgin olive oil

Sprigs of fresh basil, to garnish

FOR THE TOPPING

1 tablespoon extra virgin olive oil

1 large onion, peeled and chopped

1 green pepper, deseeded, cored and roughly chopped

8 small courgettes, trimmed and sliced about 1.25 cm thick

3 baby aubergines, roughly chopped

400 g can chopped tomatoes with garlic

1 teaspoon Herbes de Provence

Salt and pepper, to taste

Serves 4

MIXED PEPPER COUSCOUS

Couscous is made from semolina and makes a good alternative to potatoes, rice or pasta. It can be served hot or cold and is available in flavoured varieties, such as lemon and garlic. This version is infused with the aromatic juices of peppers, onions and coriander, and is delicious served with a little balsamic vinegar drizzled over it.

1 Put the dry couscous in a large mixing bowl, add the boiling water and mix briefly with a fork.

2 Stir in the olive oil and lime juice, add the chopped peppers, onion and coriander, and mix together thoroughly.

3 Leave for 30 minutes for the flavours to develop, then serve.

225 g couscous

225 ml boiling water

2 tablespoons olive oil

Juice of 1 lime

3 small peppers (green, yellow and red), deseeded and finely chopped

1 small red onion, finely chopped

80 g fresh coriander, roughly chopped

Serves 4

SPICY CHICKPEAS IN WHOLEMEAL WRAPS

FOR THE WRAPS

450 g wholewheat flour

Pinch of salt

250 ml lukewarm water

50 ml vegetable oil

FOR THE FILLING

Spray of pure vegetable oil

1 small onion, finely chopped

Small piece of fresh ginger root, peeled and grated

225 g canned tomatoes, chopped

1 green chilli, deseeded and finely chopped

½ teaspoon turmeric

2 teaspoons ground coriander

½ teaspoon garam masala

½ teaspoon chilli powder

350 g canned chickpeas, drained

FOR THE SAUCE

1 tablespoon chopped, fresh, coriander

50 ml low-fat natural yogurt

Serves 4 (makes 8 wraps)

Home-made flat bread has a wonderful flavour, and it's not at all difficult to make. It's really versatile too – you can use it as a wrap for this tasty chickpea filling, or as a flat bread, to use with dips and other accompaniments.

1   Sieve the flour and salt together. Gradually add the warm water and vegetable oil through your fingers and knead thoroughly into a stiff and pliable dough. Leave aside for half an hour to rest.

2   Heat a large saucepan and coat the base with a few sprays of oil. Add the onion and ginger, and sauté until brown. Stir in the tomatoes, green chilli, turmeric, ground coriander, garam masala and chilli powder and mix well.

3   Pour in the chickpeas and add a little water if necessary. Reduce the heat and simmer gently for 10 minutes.

4   Meanwhile, break off a piece of the dough (about the size of a walnut) and shape into a smooth ball. Flatten the ball slightly, then roll out into a circle, about 21 cm in diameter.

5   Heat a heavy-based frying pan and place the dough on the hot surface. Cook one side until brown, then turn over to cook on the other side. Finally, turn the bread again, and lightly press around the edges with a clean cloth, so that it puffs up.

6   Keep the finished breads warm by wrapping them in kitchen foil and put them to one side while you make the rest.

7   To make the serving sauce, mix the coriander leaves into the yogurt and stir thoroughly.

8   Spoon ⅛ of the chickpea mixture down the middle of each bread and carefully fold over the sides of the bread, securing with a toothpick, if necessary. Serve wraps with the yogurt sauce on the side, or with the sauce as a dip.

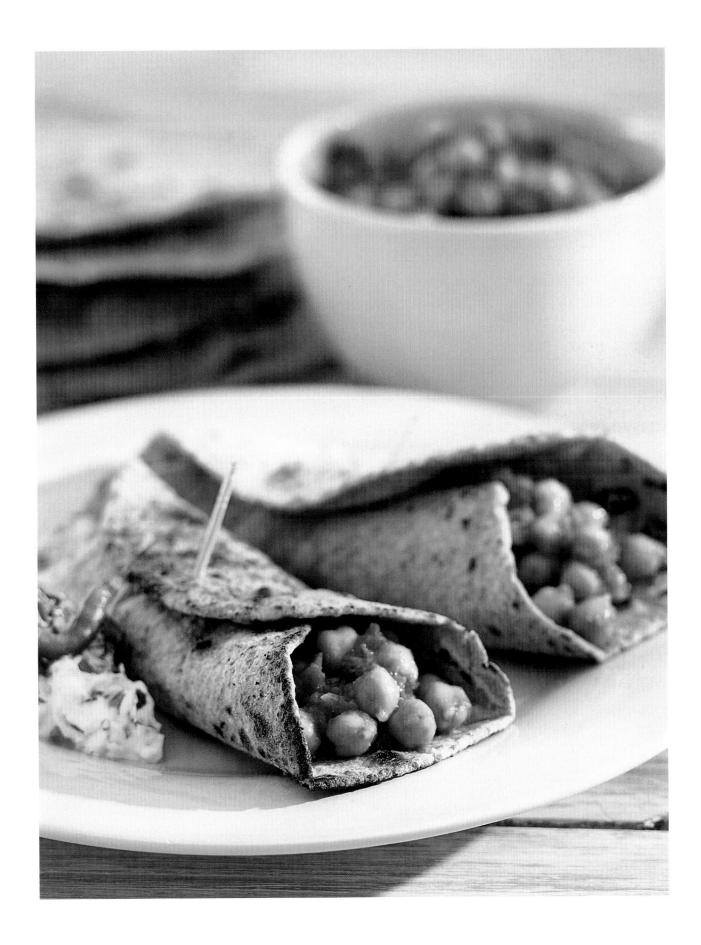

PANCAKES STUFFED WITH SPINACH & RICOTTA

FOR THE PANCAKES

200 g chickpea (gram) flour

200 ml skimmed milk

200 ml water

Pinch of salt

Spray pure vegetable oil

FOR THE FILLING

225 g baby spinach leaves

150 g ricotta cheese

¼ teaspoon nutmeg, freshly grated

25 g Parmesan cheese, grated, to serve

Fresh basil leaves, to garnish

Serves 2

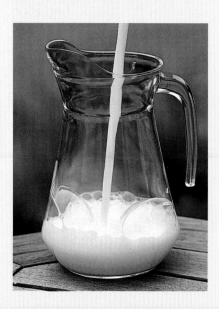

Once you've learned to make pancakes successfully, you can experiment with various different fillings. However, the spinach and ricotta combination suggested here is a true classic. Serve with a hearty mixed salad.

1 To make the pancake batter, put the chickpea flour and salt in a bowl, pour in the water and milk, and mix together thoroughly. Set aside.

2 Make the filling. Put the spinach in a saucepan without any water, and cook for about five minutes until wilted. Leave to cool slightly, drain well and chop. Add the ricotta, grate in the nutmeg and mix well. Set aside.

3 Choose a large, heavy-based frying pan, and coat with a few sprays of the oil. Place over a high heat until it is hot.

4 Remove the pan from the heat. Pour in 2–3 tablespoons of batter, tipping the frying pan as you pour it in, so that the batter covers the base.

5 Return the pan to the heat and cook for about 30 seconds until the batter has started to set on top and is golden underneath. Loosen the edges of the pancake with a thin spatula, then flip it over, and cook the other side until golden. Keep the finished pancakes warm by wrapping them in kitchen foil while you make the rest.

6 Before filling the pancakes, warm the spinach and ricotta mixture over a low heat, or heat in the microwave for 2 minutes. Fill each pancake with 2–3 tablespoons of the mixture, then fold one side over the other. Serve with a little grated Parmesan cheese and garnish with the basil leaves.

PENNE WITH ROASTED VEGETABLES

Roasted Mediterranean vegetables ooze with fragrant juices infused with the aroma of fresh garlic, giving brilliant colour and flavour to the pasta. This delicious Italian meal is a family favourite – serve it with a simple green salad and some crusty ciabatta bread.

1 Preheat the oven to 240° C, gas mark 9. Drizzle a teaspoon of oil into a large roasting tin, then layer the red and yellow peppers and courgettes into the pan, adding the herbs and seasoning in between the layers. Drizzle most of the remaining oil over the vegetables, reserving about 2 teaspoons.

2 Bake uncovered at the top of the oven for 20–25 minutes, until slightly charred, adding the tomatoes after 15 minutes. Stir once during cooking.

3 Cook the pasta in lightly salted water according to the instructions on the packet until *al dente* (around 10 minutes).

4 Meanwhile, heat the remaining oil in a large non-stick frying pan. Add the garlic, onion and green pepper and fry until the onions are light brown and the peppers are just cooked.

5 Take the vegetables out of the oven, stir gently and mix thoroughly with the pasta, adjust the seasoning if necessary, and sprinkle with parsley.

3 tablespoons olive oil

1 red pepper, diced

1 yellow pepper diced

3 medium courgettes, sliced thinly and diagonally

1½ teaspoons dried oregano

2 bay leaves

Salt and pepper to taste

3 medium tomatoes, cut into eighths

240 g dried penne

3 cloves garlic, peeled and crushed

1 small onion, finely chopped

1 green pepper, diced

1 tablespoon finely chopped fresh parsley

Serves 4

SAFFRON RICE WITH VEGETABLES & SOFT CHEESE

A colourful dish made from rice and vegetables – a perfect vegetarian meal with no need for any accompaniments. Cheese and rice contain protein and, served together, help to provide an overall balanced meal.

1 Heat the oil in a large saucepan with a lid. Fry the onions for about 5 minutes, until they are browned.

2 Add the stock, rice, vegetables, saffron and turmeric. Bring to the boil, lower the heat, cover and cook for 20 minutes, until the water is absorbed.

3 Preheat the grill to medium. Lightly grease a flameproof dish and place the cooked rice into this dish.

4 Cover the rice with a topping of low-fat soft cheese with herbs. Grill for about a minute and serve immediately.

1 tablespoon corn oil

1 medium onion, finely chopped

2 vegetable stock cubes, made up to 500 ml with boiling water

225 g long grain rice

455 g frozen mixed vegetables

Few strands of saffron

½ tsp ground turmeric

115 g low-fat soft cheese with herbs

Serves 4

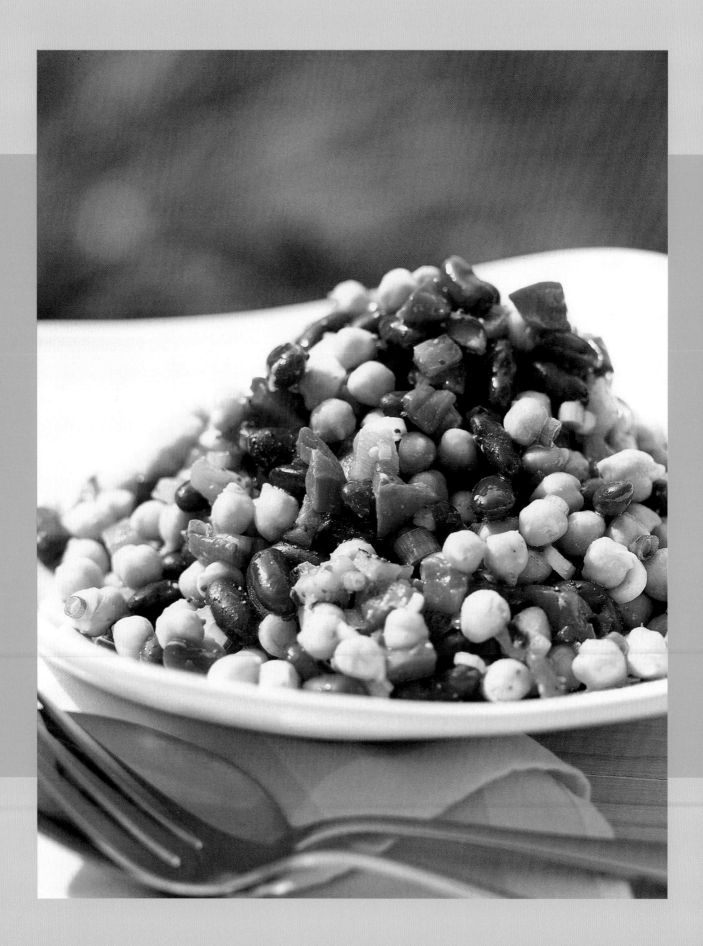

5

Vegetables & Side Dishes

POTATOES & ROOT VEGETABLES

SWEETCORN

MEDITERRANEAN VEGETABLES

PULSES & GREENS

Lemon & Onion Roasted Potatoes

600 g peeled potatoes
(about 1 kg unpeeled)

2 tablespoons olive oil

2 medium red onions, peeled and cut
into quarters

1 large lemon (or 2 small lemons), cut
into 6 wedges

Salt and pepper, to taste

Serves 4

These roast potatoes are bursting with powerful aromatic flavours and make a perfect accompaniment to grilled meat and fish.

1 Preheat the oven to 160°C, gas mark 3.

2 Cut the potatoes into equal-size pieces for roasting, and dry them thoroughly on kitchen paper.

3 Arrange the potatoes in a roasting tray and drizzle with the olive oil.

4 Add the wedges of onions and lemons and mix the vegetables together, keeping the onion pieces as whole as possible.

5 Season well. Roast for 1–1½ hours until the potatoes are crisp and golden.

Roasted New Potatoes with Tomatoes & Herbs

450 g small new potatoes in their skins,
washed and dried

1 tablespoon olive oil

2 bay leaves

2 large beef tomatoes, cut
thickly into slices

Salt and pepper, to taste

1 teaspoon fresh thyme, finely chopped
(or large pinch dried)

1 teaspoon fresh oregano, finely chopped
(or large pinch dried)

Serves 4

Baby new potatoes are just the right size for roasting in their skins, and these are deliciously scented with tomatoes and fresh herbs. They are particularly good as an accompaniment to roast lamb.

1 Preheat the oven to 190°C, gas mark 5. Cover the potatoes with boiling water and par-boil them for 3–5 minutes.

2 Make small cuts on each potato and arrange in a large roasting tin.

3 Add the olive oil, bay leaves, tomatoes, seasoning and herbs.

4 Toss roughly so that the potatoes and tomatoes are well coated, and bake in the oven for 40 minutes. Shake the tray occasionally during cooking.

ROASTED NEW POTATOES WITH HONEY & MUSTARD
After step 1, toss the par-boiled potatoes in 2 tablespoons coarse-grain mustard mixed with 2 tablespoons runny honey, and 1 tablespoon olive oil. Season to taste, and bake in the oven for 40 minutes.

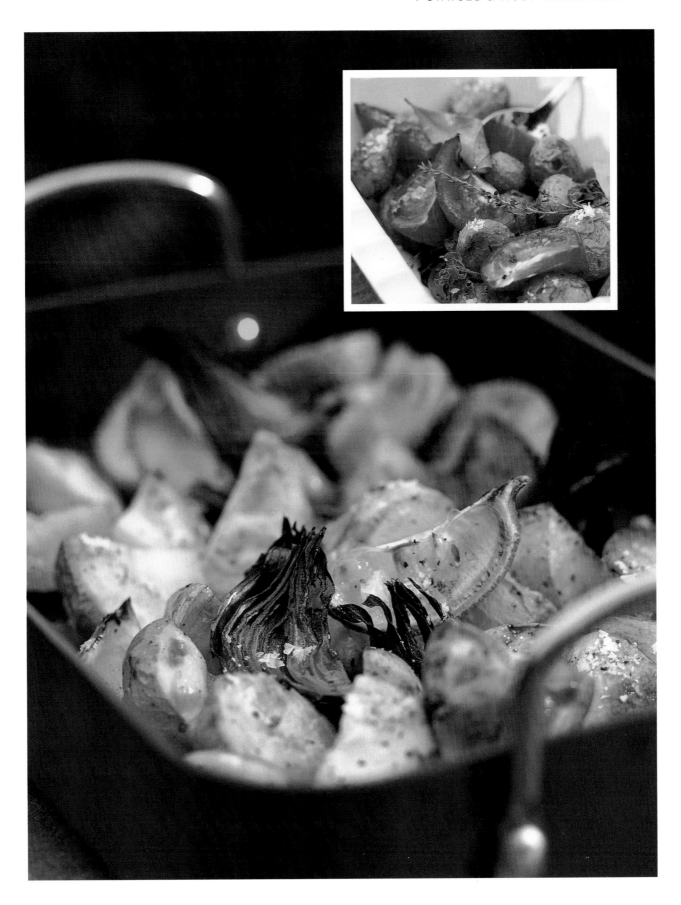

Baked Sweet Potatoes with Chilli Butter

4 sweet potatoes (each about 250–300 g)

20 g butter (or low-fat spread)

Large pinch chilli powder

Serves 4

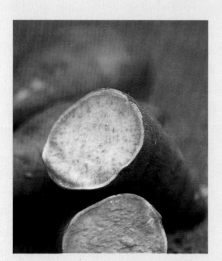

For this dish, choose sweet potatoes with orange flesh, as they have the best flavour. The potatoes ooze a sticky, delicious-tasting juice, so always roast them on a baking tray rather than a rack.

1   Preheat the oven to 200°C, gas mark 6. Wash and dry the sweet potatoes and make 2–3 deep slashes into each of them.

2   Line a baking tray with kitchen foil and arrange the sweet potatoes on it. Roast them in the oven for 40–50 minutes until they are soft.

3   Meanwhile, make the chilli butter. In a bowl, mix together the butter (or low-fat spread if using) and the chilli powder.

4   Place the mixture onto a piece of cling film, roll it into a small sausage shape then chill in the refrigerator until the potatoes are cooked.

5   When the potatoes are soft, slit them open along the top surface and spoon ¼ of the chilli butter into each one. Serve immediately.

Parsnip Croquettes

FOR THE PARSNIPS

400 g cooked potato mashed with 50 ml skimmed milk

400 g cooked parsnips, mashed

½ teaspoon ground mixed spice

FOR THE COATING

1 egg, beaten

Breadcrumbs, as required

Makes 20 croquettes

These tasty morsels have a sweeter flavour than potato croquettes, and are special enough to serve as an side dish when you're entertaining.

1   Preheat the oven to 190°C, gas mark 5.

2   In a large bowl, mix together the potato mixture, parsnips and mixed spice. Using your hands, shape the mixture into small croquettes about 4 cm long. Place the croquettes in the freezer for 5 minutes to chill.

3   Roll each croquette in the beaten egg, then in the breadcrumbs, and place in an ovenproof dish. Bake, uncovered, for 30 minutes.

SWEETCORN FRITES

These golden frites are very easy to cook, and make a tasty vegetable accompaniment to a family meal. You can vary the flavour by adding a handful of finely chopped fresh herbs or half a teaspoon of finely chopped fresh chillies.

1 Preheat the oven to 190°C, gas mark 5. Make the batter first, by sieving the flour and salt together into a large bowl. Break the egg into the middle of the flour and add the milk. Mix well, but do not beat. Leave the batter to rest in the refrigerator for 30 minutes.

2 Add the sweetcorn to the batter, and mix thoroughly.

3 Heat a heavy-based, lightly greased non-stick frying pan until it is hot and drop one tablespoon of the mixture for each fritter onto the hot surface. It is best to cook the fritters in batches of 3 or 4.

4 Bubbles will appear on the uncooked surface of each fritter. When these burst, turn the fritter over and cook the other side until it is golden brown. Brush the fritters with a little oil if they are sticking to the surface.

5 Drain them on kitchen paper to absorb any excess oil, and keep the cooked fritters warm in the oven until all of them are ready. Serve hot.

115 g plain flour

75 ml skimmed milk

¼ teaspoon salt

I large egg

325 g can sweetcorn kernels, drained

Makes 15 fritters

STIR-FRIED BABY CORN & MANGETOUT

The sesame oil and sunflower seeds add a distinctive rich, nutty flavour and crunchy texture to this crispy-fresh stir-fry.

1 Par-cook the baby corn cobs by heating them in the microwave in a little water for 3 minutes on a high setting. Alternatively, simmer them for 3 minutes in a saucepan. Drain, then cut each cob in half.

2 Heat a wok to a high temperature, then add the sesame oil. When the oil is smoking, add the mangetout, spring onions and baby corn pieces, and stir-fry for 3 minutes.

3 Sprinkle with the sunflower seeds, mix thoroughly and serve.

200 g baby corn cobs

I teaspoon sesame oil

175 g mangetout

8 spring onions, trimmed and chopped into 2 cm pieces

40 g roasted sunflower seeds

Serves 4

SESAME-FRIED GREEN BEANS
Quickly steam 455 g French beans until they are still firm but just cooked. Stir-fry 2 tablespoons of sesame seeds in 1 teaspoon of sesame oil for ½ minute, add the drained beans, cook for a few more seconds and serve immediately.

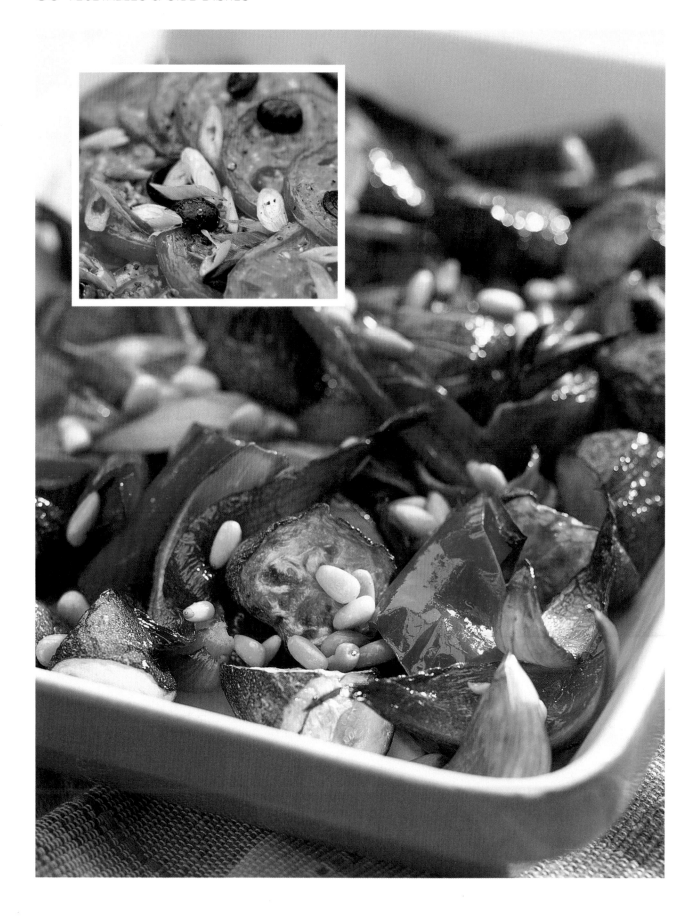

ROASTED MEDITERRANEAN VEGETABLES WITH PINE NUTS

Sweet pointed peppers are well worth tracking down at the supermarket, but if you are unable to find them, you can use bell peppers instead.

| Preheat the oven to 190°C, gas mark 5. Drizzle the olive oil into a large, oven-proof casserole dish and warm it in the oven for about 5 minutes until it is hot.

2 Add the peppers, garlic, courgettes and onion, and mix well until all the vegetables have a light coating of oil. Roast in the oven for 30–40 minutes.

3 Meanwhile, toast the pine nuts. Heat a frying pan over a medium heat and add the pine nuts. Shake the pan occasionally to move the nuts around, and toast them for 2–3 minutes until they are golden brown all over.

4 Serve the vegetables with the pine nuts sprinkled over them.

2 teaspoons olive oil

3 medium sweet, pointed red peppers, roughly chopped

4 whole garlic cloves, unpeeled

8 small courgettes, sliced

1 large red onion, peeled and chopped into large petals

55 g pine nuts

Serves 2

BAKED TOMATO & OLIVE SALAD

Tomatoes are a delicious, versatile ingredient and a good source of antioxidants. Here, they are mixed with olives, making this an ideal accompaniment to grilled fish.

| Preheat the oven to 200°C, gas mark 6. Lightly grease an oven-proof dish.

2 Layer the tomatoes and the olives into the dish, and season with the paprika and garlic salt.

3 Drizzle the olive oil over the tomatoes and olives, and bake in the middle of the oven for about 15 minutes, until the tomatoes are soft but not mushy.

4 Garnish with the spring onions and serve warm.

8 large tomatoes, sliced

12 black olives, halved

Paprika and garlic salt, to taste

1 tablespoon olive oil

2 spring onions, trimmed and finely sliced

Serves 4

Tabouleh

FOR THE SALAD

100 g bulgar wheat, pre-soaked in hot water for 1 hour, then drained

100 g flat leaf parsley, roughly chopped

5 medium tomatoes, diced

25 g leaves, finely chopped, or 2 tablespoons dried mint

1 medium onion, finely chopped

FOR THE DRESSING

Pinch salt

Pinch of ground allspice

Pinch of ground cinnamon

Juice of 2 lemons

2 tablespoons olive oil

Serves 4

This is a delightfully light, fresh-tasting salad from the Middle East. You could serve it with grilled lamb kebabs, or as an accompaniment to grilled fish.

1　In a bowl, mix together the wheat, parsley, tomatoes, mint and onions.

2　Make the dressing. Put all the dressing ingredients into a screw-top jar, cover and shake vigorously.

3　Toss the wheat mixture in the dressing, and serve.

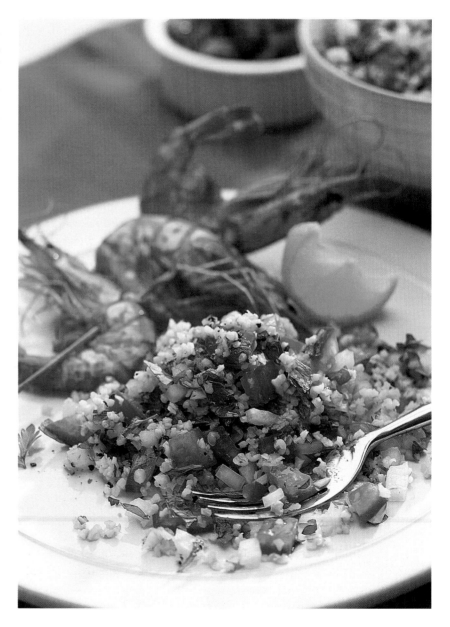

PEPPERY BEAN SALAD

This colourful salad is packed with flavour, and goes well with grilled fish; alternatively, it could make a delicious vegetarian dish – serve it with warmed pitta bread to mop up the fragrant dressing.

1 Preheat the grill. Place the peppers skin side up on the grill tray, and cook under a high heat for about 15 minutes, or until the skins are blackened. Put them inside a plastic bag, and leave to cool for 10 minutes.

2 Peel the peppers, then dice and place in a large bowl. Add the spring onions, kidney beans and chickpeas and mix.

3 Put all the dressing ingredients into a screw-top jar, and shake vigorously. Pour the dressing over the salad, and mix well.

4 Cover with cling film and chill for at least 15 minutes before serving.

FOR THE SALAD

1 red pepper, halved and deseeded

1 green pepper, halved and deseeded

4 spring onions, trimmed and finely chopped

200 g can red kidney beans, drained

400 g can chickpeas, drained

FOR THE DRESSING

1½ tablespoons olive oil

Juice of 1 small lemon

1 clove garlic, peeled and crushed

2 teaspoons wholegrain French mustard

Serves 4

CABBAGE WITH CARAWAY SEEDS

Lightly steamed, and scattered with delicately flavoured caraway seeds, this is the perfect way to prepare cabbage. Serve it with griddled lamb chops, or thin slices of roast beef.

1 Steam the cabbage for 2–3 minutes until it is just cooked, but still a little firm. Drain thoroughly.

2 Heat the oil in a wok until it is smoking, add the cabbage, caraway seeds and seasoning and stir-fry for 2–3 minutes. Sprinkle on some cayenne pepper and serve immediately.

455 g white cabbage, sliced

1 tablespoon olive oil

2 tablespoons caraway seeds

Salt and pepper, to taste

Pinch of cayenne pepper

Serves 4

RED CABBAGE COLESLAW

The reduced-calorie mayonnaise in this side dish helps to keep the fat lower than in a standard coleslaw. If you want it even lower in fat, choose a low-fat natural yogurt or fat-free vinaigrette instead.

Simply mix all the ingredients together in a bowl and serve. If you are not eating this immediately, cover the bowl and keep it in the refrigerator until it is ready to serve.

225 g red cabbage, shredded or grated

3 medium carrots, grated

3 spring onions, trimmed and sliced

115 ml low-calorie mayonnaise

Serves 4

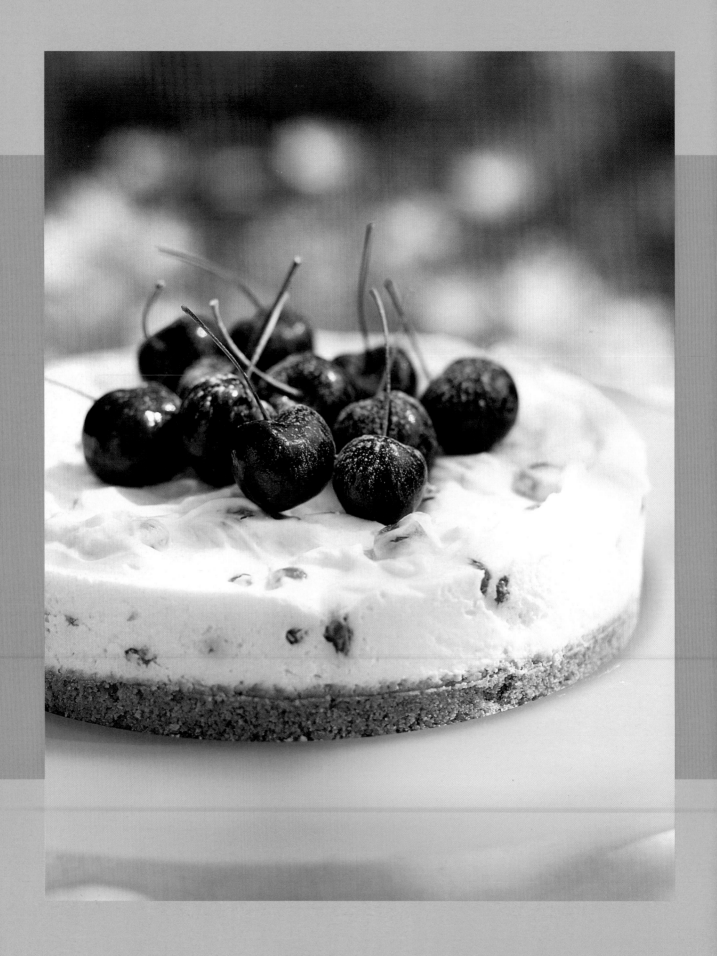

6 Desserts

RASPBERRY SOUFFLE OMELETTE

Here's a deliciously simple dessert with a light, fluffy texture. The hint of almond essence adds an aromatic touch.

2 large eggs at room temperature, separated

25 g caster sugar

2–3 drops almond essence

2 teaspoons oil

I tablespooon warmed pure fruit raspberry spread

8 fresh raspberries, halved and 2 teaspoons sifted icing sugar, to serve

Serves 2

1 Whisk the egg yolks with the caster sugar and almond essence until they are light and fluffy.

2 With a clean, dry whisk, whisk the egg whites stiffly in a dry bowl and mix them lightly with the egg yolks and sugar.

3 Preheat the grill to high. Heat the oil in a non-stick omelette pan, pour in the omelette mixture and cook for about 2–3 minutes until it is just set.

4 Cook the omelette under the grill for about a minute until it is browned.

5 Quickly spread with warmed jam, fold over and tip onto a warm plate.

6 Decorate with fresh raspberries and icing sugar and serve immediately.

BAKED BANANAS WITH ORANGE

Baked bananas are naturally sweet, and these are given a refreshing citrus tang with the juice, zest and peel of orange. This is a lovely dessert for winter evenings, as it is both warming and light. Serve it on its own, or with a scoop of reduced-fat ice cream.

4 medium bananas

2 tablespoons unsweetened orange juice

Zest of one orange

30 g dried orange peel

Serves 4

1 Preheat the oven to 220°C, gas mark 7. Make a lengthways slit in each banana, taking care that the skin doesn't peel off.

2 Cut four 30 cm x 30 cm square pieces of kitchen foil, and place one banana in each. Pour the juice and zest into each slit.

3 Sprinkle each banana with the dried peel and wrap in a foil parcel, sealing with a double fold on the top and ends, leaving space for steam to expand.

4 Place the foil parcels on a non-stick baking tray and bake in the oven for 15–20 minutes until the bananas are soft.

CHARRED FRUIT KEBABS

Enjoy a mouth-watering feast of tangy grilled fruits coated with a mix of honey and lime juice. In the summer months, you can cook these on an outdoor barbecue. If you're using wooden skewers, remember to soak them in water first. Serve with low-fat natural yogurt.

1 Preheat the grill and line the tray with foil. Place the fruit in a bowl.

2 Mix the lime juice with the honey and stir into the fruit, making sure that the chunks are coated well on all sides.

3 Thread the chunks of fruit alternately onto four skewers and grill for about 5 minutes until softened.

I mango, peeled, pitted and cut into bite-sized chunks

½ small pineapple, cored and cut into bite-sized chunks

2 kiwi fruit, peeled and quartered

I tablespoon lime juice

2 teaspoons runny honey

Serves 4

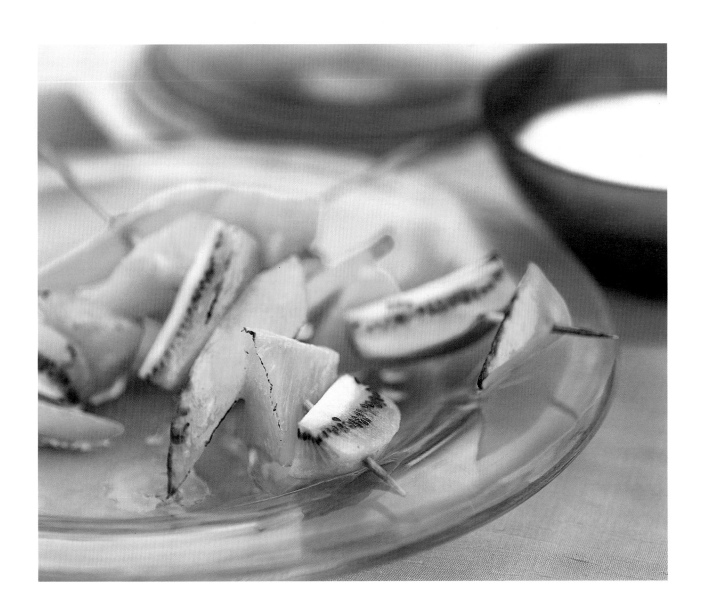

AMARETTO & ALMOND STUFFED PEACHES

Almond flavours add their intensely aromatic note to the sweet ripeness of the peaches in this simple but elegant dish. Peach halves canned in natural juice are an excellent substitute if you don't have fresh ones. The butter is necessary to achieve the right texture, but very little is used, so you can indulge with a clear conscience.

4 very ripe fresh peaches, or 8 peach halves, canned in natural juice and drained

FOR THE STUFFING

25 g ground almonds

15 g soft butter

25 g caster sugar

2 tablespoons Amaretto liqueur or other almond liqueur

100 g half-fat crème fraîche, to serve

Serves 4

1 Preheat the oven to 190°C, gas mark 5.

2 If you're using canned, drained peaches, go to step 3. If you're using fresh peaches, put them into a bowl of boiling water. Leave for 1 minute, then peel off the skins. Cut through to the stones lengthways, then twist sharply to separate the two halves. Remove the stones and any fibrous tissue.

3 Mix the almonds with the butter, sugar and liqueur and use this mixture to stuff the peach halves.

4 Arrange the peaches on a lightly greased baking tray, stuffing side up and bake in the centre of the oven for 15 minutes.

5 Serve warm or cold with a swirl of crème fraîche.

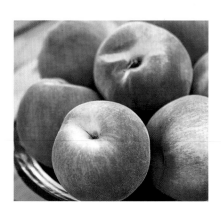

POACHED PEARS WITH FRUIT COULIS

This deceptively simple dessert has an exquisite flavour and needs no added sugar. It tastes particularly delicious if you use a ripe, naturally sweet pear, such as Blush Rosada. The pears will look even more spectacular if they are left whole – preferably with the stems on, though the poaching time will take about five minutes longer.

4 ripe pears, halved lengthwise and cores removed

Juice of 1 lemon

FOR THE FRUIT COULIS

225 g forest fruits or raspberries, (thawed if frozen)

Sprig of fresh redcurrants, to decorate

Serves 4

1 Arrange the pears in a large shallow-based pan, with the cored side facing down, in a single layer.

2 Mix the lemon juice with enough cold water to cover the pears. Bring to the boil, lower the heat and simmer gently for 5–10 minutes. The timing depends on the variety and the ripeness of the pears that you use. They should remain quite firm, but soft enough to get a dessert fork through.

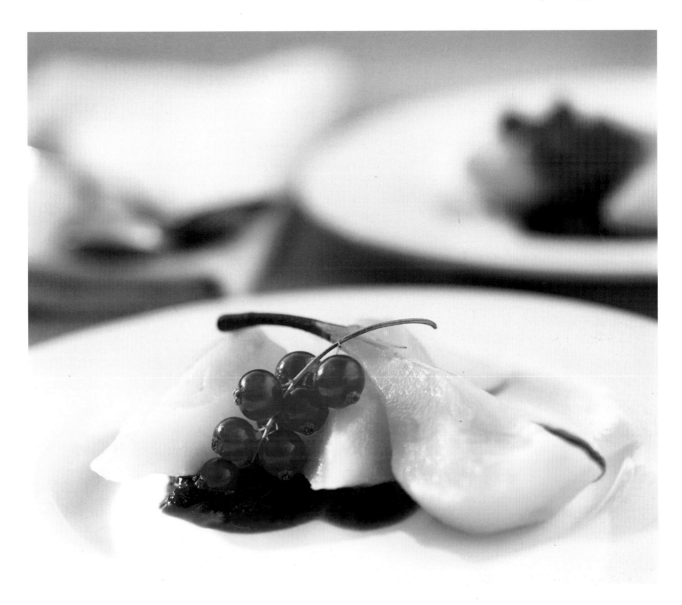

3   Transfer the poached pears to 4 serving plates and leave aside to cool.

4   Meanwhile, make the coulis. Purée the forest fruits or raspberries in a
    blender or food processor, then push the mixture through a fine sieve in
    order to remove the pips.

5   Spoon or pipe the coulis around the pear halves and decorate with a sprig
    of fresh redcurrants before serving.

WHOLESOME BREAD & BUTTER PUDDING

4 slices wholemeal bread

40 g softened half-fat butter

25 g caster sugar

55 g sultanas

3 medium eggs

350 ml skimmed milk

½ teaspoon freshly-grated nutmeg

Serves 4

If you have some leftover stale bread, you can use it to make this wonderfully comforting dessert. Any variety of brown bread is fine, although wholemeal gives a lighter result than stone-ground. You can also use currants or raisins instead of sultanas.

1 Preheat the oven to 180°C, gas mark 4. Butter each slice of bread with the butter, saving a little to grease the baking dish.

2 Grease a 1 litre baking dish. Cut each slice in half diagonally, leaving the crusts on, and arrange in the dish in alternating layers, each layer sprinkled with the sugar and sultanas.

3 Whisk the eggs and milk together then strain over the bread mixture. Leave to stand for at least 15–20 minutes, until well soaked.

4 Sprinkle with the grated nutmeg and bake for 35–40 minutes until the pudding is risen and golden. A knife inserted in the centre should come out clean. Serve warm.

APPLE & PLUM CRUMBLE

85 g wholewheat flour

100 g porridge oats

25 g reduced-fat margarine, chilled and diced

55 g soft brown sugar

5 medium ripe plums, halved and stoned

2 large dessert apples, peeled and sliced

1 teaspoon powdered cinnamon

2 tablespoons water

Serves 4

This is a favourite traditional dessert, and is both wholesome and warming. You can experiment with different combinations of fruit, such as apple and rhubarb or apricot and banana. Serve hot with a low-fat custard or half-fat crème fraîche.

1 Preheat the oven to 180°C, gas mark 4.

2 Put the flour and oats into a large bowl, add the margarine and rub it in lightly with your fingertips until the mixture resembles coarse crumbs.

3 Stir in half the sugar and mix well.

4 Arrange the plums and apple slices in a lightly greased pie dish. Sprinkle on the remainder of the sugar and the cinnamon, then add the water.

5 Now sprinkle on the crumble mixture, smoothing it over with a fork.

6 Bake above the centre of the oven for 35 minutes or until top is golden brown. Serve hot or warm.

BLACK FOREST CRÊPES

These are equally delicious made with any variety of jam, but cherry conserve adds the authentic Black Forest touch. If crêpes are a favourite dessert, it's worth making a double batch and freezing them between sheets of baking parchment, ready to be defrosted and filled.

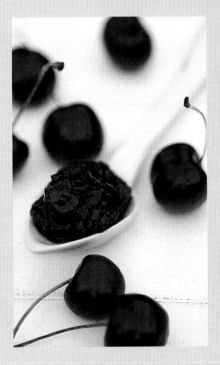

1 Sift the flour and salt into a large bowl. Make a well in the centre of the mixture and break in the egg.

2 Add a little milk and beat with a balloon whisk, gradually adding a little more milk at a time, until a smooth batter is formed.

3 Beat for 1–2 more minutes until the surface of the batter is covered with tiny bubbles, then leave to stand for 30 minutes.

4 Brush the base of a non-stick omelette pan with the oil. Heat until sizzling, then pour in one eighth of the batter, swirling it around to cover the base of the pan.

5 Cook for 1–2 minutes until the underside of the crêpe is golden. Using a plastic spatula, loosen the crêpe, flip it over, and cook for a further 1–2 minutes. Transfer to a warm plate, and cover with baking parchment.

6 Brush the pan with a little more oil and repeat the cooking process for the remainder of the crêpes, stacking them between layers of parchment.

7 When they are ready to serve, spread each crêpe with the black cherry conserve (or reduced-sugar jam) and roll it up.

8 Allow 2 pancakes per serving and decorate them with a swirl of crème fraîche and a dusting of grated chocolate.

FRESH STRAWBERRY CRÊPES

For a lower calorie alternative, pile 200 g fresh strawberry halves and 125 g Greek yoghurt into the crêpes instead of the jam and crème fraîche. Scatter over some passion fruit seeds in place of the chocolate.

FOR THE CRÊPES

115 g plain flour

Pinch of salt

1 large egg

300 ml skimmed milk

2 teaspoons sunflower oil

FOR THE FILLING

100 g low-sugar black cherry conserve, or reduced-sugar blackcurrant jam

115 g half-fat crème fraîche and 25 g dark chocolate, grated, to decorate

Serves 4 (makes 8 crêpes)

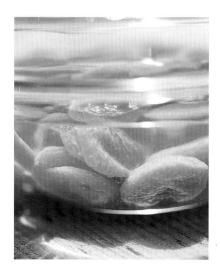

2 teaspoons sunflower oil

100 g soft dark brown sugar

1 teaspoon powdered cinnamon

250 g dried apricots, soaked overnight and drained

FOR THE PASTRY

55 g plain white flour

55 g plain wholemeal flour

Pinch of salt

55 g chilled reduced-fat spread

2–3 tablespoons water

Serves 6

APRICOT & APPLE TARTE TATIN

A tarte tatin is a French classic – an upside-down tart with the pastry baked on top of the fruit, then, after it has been baked, inverted to serve. This recipe uses wholemeal flour and dried apricots, but you can use white flour and ready-to-eat apricots if you prefer. Caramelised brown sugar adds a sweet crunch of delicious indulgence.

1 Preheat the oven to 180°C, gas mark 4.

2 To make the pastry, sift the plain and wholemeal flours and the salt into a bowl, adding any bran left behind in the sieve. Cut the spread into into small pieces, and rub it in with your fingertips until the mixture has the texture of fine breadcrumbs. Mix in enough cold water to form a soft dough, then wrap in cling film and chill for 30 minutes.

3 Prepare the upside-down topping. Brush a 20 cm cake tin with half of the sunflower oil. Cut a circle of baking parchment to fit the base, grease it with the remainder of the oil and place it into the base of the tin.

4 Coat the parchment with the sugar, pressing it down firmly and evenly.

5 Sprinkle with the cinnamon and arrange the apricots on top, again pressing them down firmly and evenly.

6 Roll out the dough on a lightly-floured board and cut out a circle to fit on top of the apricots, pressing down gently. Chill for 15–20 minutes.

7 Bake for 40 minutes or until the pastry is golden.

8 Allow to cool, loosen lightly round the edges with a spatula, and invert the tart onto a large plate. Remove the baking parchment before serving.

CHILLED LEMON & LIME MOUSSE

The clean citrus tang of lemon and lime add refreshing zest to this classic dessert. You can use lemons or limes on their own, but a combination of the two is spectacular. This mousse does have the richness of whipped cream and sugar, though the soft cheese used is a lower fat version. It is delicious with low sugar shortbread (see page 117). All in all, a refreshing creamy dessert which has all the freshness of citrus fruits and a touch of Grand Marnier just to make it even more special.

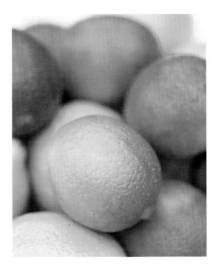

1   Whisk the cheese using an electric whisk until it is light and fluffy.

2   Add the icing sugar, lemon juice, lime juice, food colouring (if using) and whipped cream and continue to whisk until the mixture is soft and creamy.

3   Fold in the Grand Marnier and spoon into individual glasses or sundae dishes.

4   Decorate each dish with mint leaves and topping of your choice, see below. Chill in the refrigerator.

225 g lower fat soft cheese

100 g icing sugar

Juice of 2 lemons

Juice of 2 limes

2–3 drops food colouring (optional)

150 ml whipping cream, whipped

1 tablespoon Grand Marnier

Few fresh mint leaves

Serves 4

MOUSSE TOPPINGS

A complementary garnish would be 4 slices each of crystallised lemon and lime, each cut in half. Alternatively, you could use a tablespoon of mixed lemon and lime peel, which is sold shredded. For a fresh fruit alternative, a few black grapes or slices of mandarin placed on top of each mousse will make an attractive contrast.

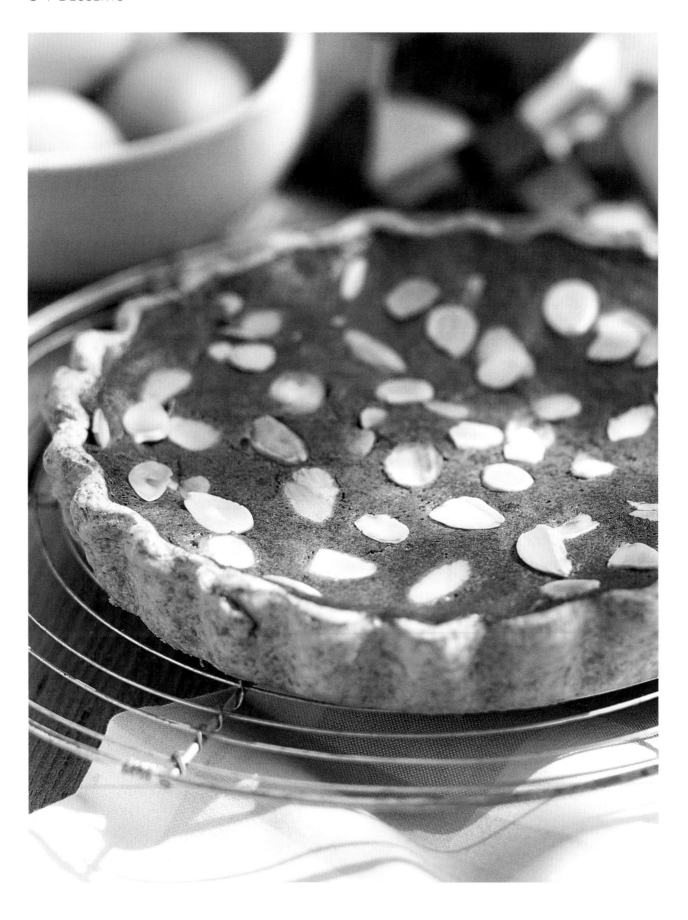

CHOCOLATE & ALMOND CUSTARD TART

This tart is made with an old-fashioned egg custard filling. It is relatively high in fat, so reserve it for special occasions. Always use reduced-fat spread, as lower-fat varieties are too high in water for successful pastry-making.

1 Preheat the oven to 180°C, gas mark 4. Sift the plain and wholemeal flours and the salt into a bowl, adding any bran left behind in the sieve.

2 Cut the spread into into small pieces, and rub it in with your fingertips until the mixture has the texture of fine breadcrumbs. Mix in enough cold water to form a soft dough, wrap in cling film and chill for 30 minutes.

3 Roll out the dough and use it to line a 20 cm flan tin.

4 Line the pastry shell with kitchen foil or baking parchment, and fill it with dried beans, uncooked rice or ceramic baking beans. Place in the oven to bake blind for 10 minutes. Remove from the oven, discard the foil or paper and beans (if using) and bake for a further 5 minutes. Leave to cool.

5 Meanwhile, whisk the eggs and sugar together in a bowl until they are light and fluffy.

6 Put the milk, chocolate and vanilla essence into a small saucepan and heat gently, stirring continuously, until the chocolate has completely melted and blended in with the milk. Do not allow the milk to boil.

7 Pour into the beaten eggs, mix well, then strain into the pastry case and top with the flaked almonds. Bake for 30–40 minutes until the pastry is golden and the custard has just set.

8 Cool on a wire rack before serving.

FOR THE PASTRY

55 g plain white flour

55 g plain wholemeal flour

Pinch of salt

55 g chilled reduced-fat spread

2–3 tablespoons water

FOR THE FILLING

2 medium eggs, lightly beaten

25 g caster sugar

225 ml skimmed milk

50g good quality dark chocolate (75% cocoa solids), broken into small pieces

2–3 drops vanilla essence

2 tablespoons flaked almonds, to decorate

Serves 8

CINNAMON CUSTARD TART
Omit the chocolate and make the egg custard as above. Add a level teaspoon of ground cinnamon, the zest of half a lemon, a few drops of vanilla essence and some grated nutmeg. Dust with cinnamon before serving.

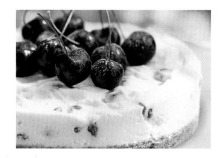

Lemon & Sultana Cheesecake with Cherries

Cheesecake is generally high in fat and calories when made with full-fat soft cheese and fresh cream. But you can go ahead and enjoy this feather-light American-style version, as the filling is virtually fat-free. For a spectacular topping, use very ripe black cherries.

FOR THE BISCUIT BASE

175 g crushed digestive biscuits

55 g reduced-fat spread, very soft

FOR THE TOPPING

2 sachets (11 g sachets) powdered gelatine, dissolved in a little orange juice

Juice of 1 lemon

350 g skimmed milk soft cheese or fromage frais

115 g low-fat natural yogurt

55 g granulated sugar

55 g sultanas

115 g very ripe black cherries

2 teaspoons icing sugar

Serves 8

1 Mix the biscuits thoroughly with the spread. Press firmly into the base of a 20 cm loose-bottomed cake tin and chill for 1 hour or until firm.

2 Meanwhile put the dissolved gelatine into a blender or food processor along with the lemon juice, cheese, yoghurt and sugar.

3 Blend for a few seconds and transfer to a large bowl. Mix in the sultanas.

4 Pour onto the biscuit-crumb base and chill. After about 2 hours, or when just beginning to firm up, place the icing sugar in a little sieve and shake over the cherries. Place the sugared cherries on top of the cake.

5 Return to fridge and chill until completely set.

Petits Coeurs à La Crème

Traditionally this classic French dessert is made in small, perforated heart-shaped moulds – hence the name petits coeurs. You can get the moulds from specialist kitchenware suppliers, but alternatively, you can use one large colander or sieve. The recipe benefits from being lower in fat and sugar than the classic version, as skimmed milk soft cheese and low-fat yogurt replace the traditionally richer ingredients.

250 g skimmed milk soft cheese

55 g low-fat natural yoghurt

2 tablespoons semi-skimmed milk

1 teaspoon vanilla or almond essence

40 g sieved caster sugar

225 g strawberries or raspberries

4 small sprigs mint leaves

Serves 4

1 Process the cheese, yogurt and milk in a blender or food processor until smooth, then transfer to a mixing bowl.

2 Add the essence and sugar and mix thoroughly.

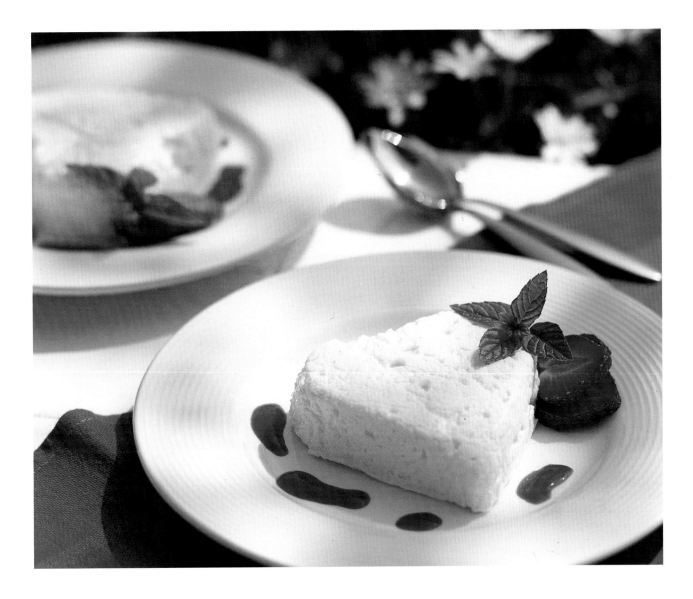

3 Spoon into 4 small perforated moulds or 1 large one (see introduction above), lined with damp muslin and carefully smooth the tops.

4 Stand on a wire rack over a baking tin or tray and leave to drain for 6–8 hours in a refrigerator.

5 Meanwhile, purée the berries in a blender or food processor, reserving 4 berries for the garnish.

6 To serve, turn out and encircle with the strawberry purée. Garnish with fresh mint sprigs and the reserved strawberries, cut into halves.

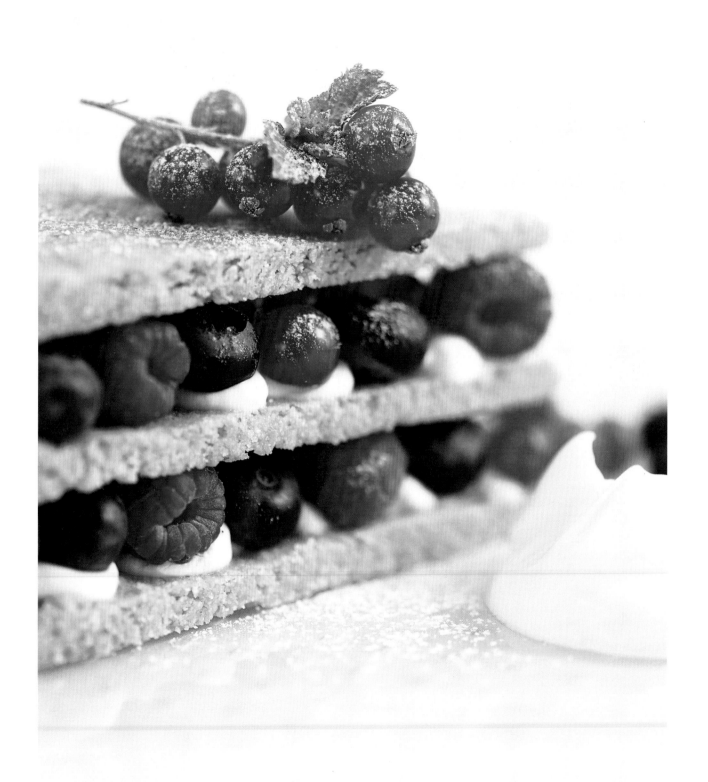

RASPBERRY & BLUEBERRY SHORTCAKE STACKS

These American style shortcake treats are simple to make and surprisingly rich, despite the sneaky low-fat crème fraîche. The shortcake is crunchy and crumbly – make sure you work the mixture well into the corners of the tin, making the surface as even as possible and mark out the divisions deeply before baking.

1 Preheat the oven to 150°C, gas mark 2. Lightly grease and line a 20 cm square cake tin with non-stick baking parchment.

2 Cream the butter and sugar together until light and fluffy.

3 Sift in the flour and add the ground rice, a little at a time, mixing steadily with a wooden spoon. Use your fingers to make a smooth but firm dough.

4 Press gently into the prepared tin, making sure you distribute the mixture evenly and flatly. Cut right the way through into 12 squares.

5 Bake for 55 minutes or until the shortcake is firm and lightly browned. Remove from the tin, gently break into 12 pieces and allow to cool.

6 When you are ready to serve, top four of the shortcake squares with half the berries and half the crème fraîche.

7 Add four more squares on top and then add a layer of the remaining berries and crème fraîche.

8 Finally, lay the last four squares on top, and decorate with a sprig of redcurrants. Sieve the icing sugar and sprinkle about a teaspoon of icing sugar onto each stack.

FOR THE SHORTBREAD

85 g butter

35 g caster sugar

100 g plain white flour

70 g ground rice

FOR THE FILLING

55 g fresh raspberries

55 g fresh blueberries

4 tablespoons half-fat crème fraîche

FOR THE TOPPING

Sprig of redcurrants

4 teaspoons icing sugar

Serves 4

Raspberry & Ginger Sundaes

This is such an easy dessert to make, yet it tastes really good. Spicy ginger, sweet raspberries and creamy crème fraîche make a gratifying blend of flavours and contrasting textures.

FOR THE BISCUIT BASE

175 g ginger biscuits, crushed

55 g reduced-fat spread, melted

FOR THE TOPPING

225 g half-fat crème fraîche

2 small pieces stem ginger, finely chopped

3 tablespoons granulated sweetener

300 g fresh raspberries

Serves 4

1 Mix the crushed biscuits with the reduced-fat spread and spoon into 4 individual trifle or sundae dishes. Chill for 30 minutes, or until firm.

2 Mix the crème fraîche with the chopped ginger and 2 tablespoons of the sweetener, then spoon it over each crushed biscuit base.

3 Top with the raspberries, sprinkle over the remainder of the sweetener and chill again before serving.

Exotic Fruit Salad with Cardamom

This luscious salad is made from an exotic mix of fruits scented with cardamom. You can use any combination of fruit you like, but the secret is to have a variety of colours and textures. Serve with a final swirl of half-fat crème fraîche for creamy contrast.

FOR THE SYRUP

55 g granulated sugar

Zest of 1 lemon

8 green cardamom pods, cracked slightly, but still retaining their seeds

300 ml water

2 large mangoes, skin and stone removed and cut into cubes

2 bananas, peeled and sliced

2 papaya, peeled and diced

1 large red apple, cut into quarters, core removed and sliced (leave skin on)

2 small red pears, prepared in the same way as the apple above

Serves 6–8

1 First make the syrup. Place the granulated sugar in a saucepan with the lemon zest and cardamom. Add the water and heat until boiling, then lower the heat and simmer for 2 minutes.

2 Remove from the heat, add a couple of ice cubes to cool the syrup, then pour it into a large bowl.

3 As you prepare the fruit, add it to the syrup immediately, and mix together well. Otherwise the fruit will go brown with exposure to the air.

4 Cover and place in the refrigerator for at least 1 hour before serving so that the flavours have time to mingle.

5 Remove the cardamom pods before you serve (the seeds are edible).

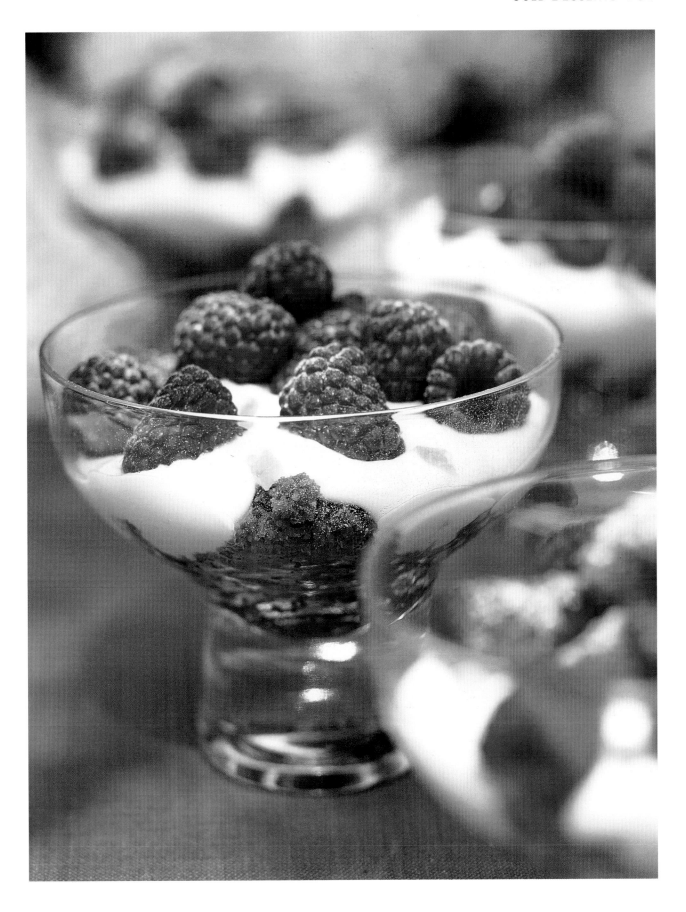

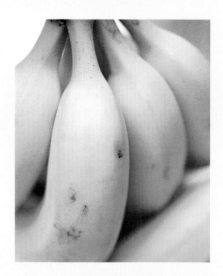

Banana Ice Cream with Chocolate & Hazelnut Topping

This home-made ice cream is a special treat, mingling the sweet flavours of bananas and chocolate with the satisfying crunch of hazelnuts. Serve this dessert after a high fibre main meal, to slow down the absorption of its sugar. Remember to turn the freezer or freezer compartment of your refrigerator to its coldest setting at least 1 hour before starting.

FOR THE ICE CREAM

3 large ripe bananas, peeled and coarsely chopped

Juice of 1 lemon

1 x 410 g can reduced-fat evaporated milk, chilled

1 tablespoon caster sugar

FOR THE TOPPING

100 g dark chocolate

2 tablespoons water

15 g half-fat spread

50 g hazelnuts, coarsely chopped

Serves 4

1   Mash the bananas in a large bowl until thick and pulpy. Add the lemon juice and mash again.

2   In a separate bowl, whip the evaporated milk with an electric or rotary hand beater until it is thick and frothy and almost doubled in volume.

3   Add this to the pulped bananas, a little at a time, beating continuously until it is thick and smooth. Stir in the sugar.

4   Pour into a pre-chilled rigid polythene container, cover and freeze for 1 hour or until just beginning to set round the edges.

5   Whisk thoroughly until smooth, re-cover and freeze again for 2–3 hours, checking after two hours, until frozen through.

6   Meanwhile, make the topping. Break the chocolate into squares and put it into a small pan with the water. Suspend over a larger pan of gently simmering water and stir until completely melted. Remove from the heat and beat in the half-fat spread. Allow to cool, and stir in the chopped hazelnuts.

7   Move the ice cream to the main body of the refrigerator for 30 minutes before serving. Pour the sauce over the ice cream just before serving.

SUMMER BERRY FROZEN DESSERT

You can use any mixture of summer berries for this, but it's a good idea to include blackcurrants or blackberries, as they give a gloriously rich colour. You can also use frozen fruits, but make sure they are thawed and drained before blending. Turn the freezer or freezer compartment of your refrigerator to its coldest setting at least 1 hour before you start.

1 Put the fruit into a blender or food processor with the sugar and blend for about 1 minute until it is puréed.

2 Rub the purée through a nylon sieve to remove any pips, then mix in the lemon juice and yogurt.

3 Pour the mixture into a pre-chilled rigid polythene container, cover and freeze for 1 hour until it is half solidified.

4 Whisk until the mixture is smooth and creamy, cover and freeze again for 3 hours, checking after two hours, until frozen through.

5 Move the dessert to the main body of the refrigerator 30 minutes before serving and decorate it with the whole raspberries.

115 g each of raspberries, strawberries and blackcurrants or frozen summer fruits

55 g granulated sugar

1 teaspoon lemon juice

225 g low-fat natural yogurt

25 g raspberries, to decorate

Serves 4

STRAWBERRY & MASCARPONE SORBET

This sorbet is a particularly refreshing summer dessert. Though sorbets can be a time-consuming dessert to make, the delicious combination of the creamy Italian cheese and the fresh strawberries make the extra effort worthwhile.

1 Put the strawberries into a processor or blender, and blend with the sugar and lemon juice for about 1 minute.

2 Beat the soft cheese with the yogurt, then mix in the strawberry purée. Spoon the mixture into a pre-chilled rigid polythene container. Cover and freeze for about 1 hour until crystals start to form around the edges.

3 Whisk briskly, return to the freezer and repeat this stage 2 or 3 times until the sorbet is smooth and completely frozen through.

4 Scoop into long-stemmed glasses and serve garnished with strawberries and fresh mint.

300 g fresh strawberries, hulled

75 g caster sugar

1 tablespoon lemon juice

155 g mascarpone cheese

115 g thick Greek yogurt

Fresh strawberries and fresh mint leaves, to serve

Serves 4

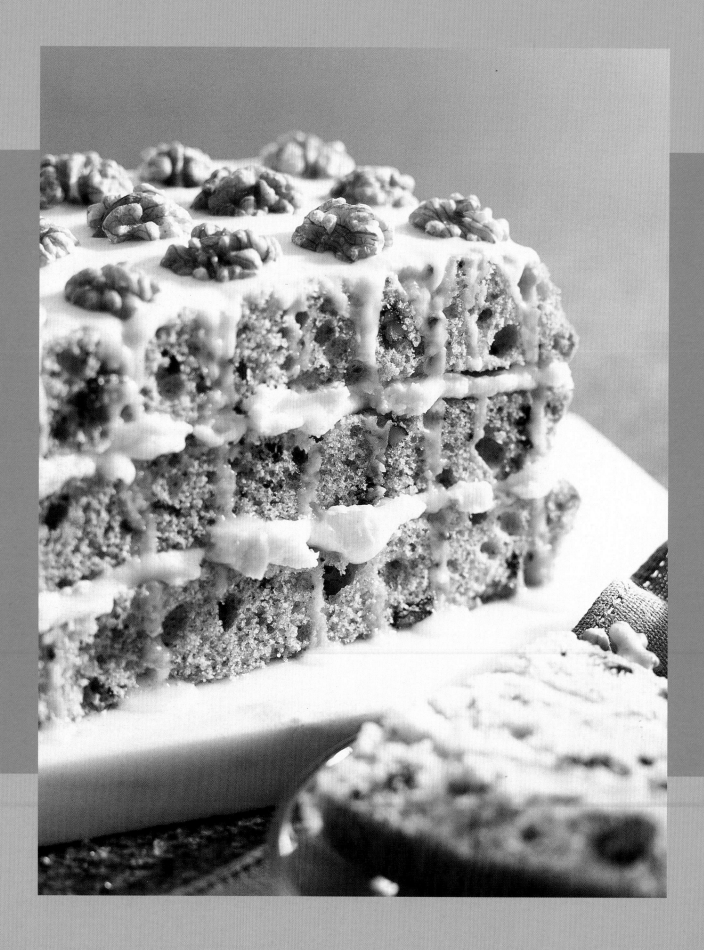

7

Cakes,
Cookies &
Breads

FRUIT SCONES

115 g self-raising white flour

115 g wholewheat flour

2 teaspoons baking powder

Pinch of salt

40 g polyunsaturated margarine (at room temperature)

25 g caster sugar

55 g sultanas

150 ml skimmed milk (keep 2 teaspoons on one side for brushing the tops of the scones before baking)

Makes 12

Freshly made scones are a real treat – and these are so easy to make. Serve them simply with low-fat spread, or indulge yourself and smother them in low-fat fromage frais, fresh strawberries and a sprinkling of chopped nuts or flaked chocolate. You could use all white flour or all wholewheat, but the 50/50 mixture used here works well and provides a healthy balance without being too heavy.

1   Preheat the oven to 220°C, gas mark 7. Sift the self-raising and wholewheat flour into a bowl with the baking powder and salt, tipping any left over bran into the sifted mixture.

2   Lightly rub in the margarine with fingertips until the mixture has the consistency of fine breadcrumbs.

3   Mix in the sugar and sultanas (the same quantities of dried mixed peel or chopped glace cherries can be used instead) and add the milk a little at a time, mixing well with a palette knife until a soft dough is formed.

4   Turn out onto a lightly-floured board and roll out to a thickness of 2 cm. Using a 4 cm pastry cutter, cut out the scones, re-rolling the leftover dough as necessary until you have used it all.

5   Place the scones on a lightly-greased baking sheet, brush the tops with a little skimmed milk to glaze, and bake near the top of the oven for 15–20 minutes until golden.

6   Cool on a wire rack until the scones are just warm, then serve.

GRANDMA'S HOME-MADE GINGERBREAD

This old fashioned cake fills the kitchen with delicious spicy aromas while it is baking. Be sure to use reduced-fat spread – low-fat versions contain more water and do not give good results. As this gingerbread won't keep well for more than 2–3 days, you might want to freeze some for later.

1 Preheat the oven to 180°C, gas mark 4.

2 Lightly grease a square, shallow 20 cm cake tin and line it with non-stick baking parchment.

3 Sift the flour and bicarbonate of soda and mix with the sugar, cinnamon, ginger and sultanas.

4 In a large bowl, cream the reduced-fat spread with the treacle, then mix in the flour and fruit mixture.

5 Add the beaten egg and milk, mixing thoroughly to a fairly stiff, but not runny, consistency.

6 Spoon the mixture into the greased and lined tin and bake for 25 minutes.

7 Reduce the oven temperature to 160°C, gas mark 3 and continue baking for 25–35 minutes, or until a skewer inserted into the centre comes out clean.

8 Cool in the tin for 15 minutes, then turn out and leave to cool completely on a wire rack. Cut into 16 squares before serving.

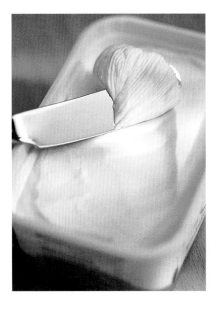

280 g plain flour

1 teaspoon bicarbonate of soda

Pinch salt

55 g soft dark brown sugar

2 teaspoons ground cinnamon

2 teaspoons ground ginger

175 g sultanas

115 g reduced-fat spread at room temperature

85 g black treacle

1 large egg, beaten

150 ml skimmed milk, just warm

Makes 16 slices

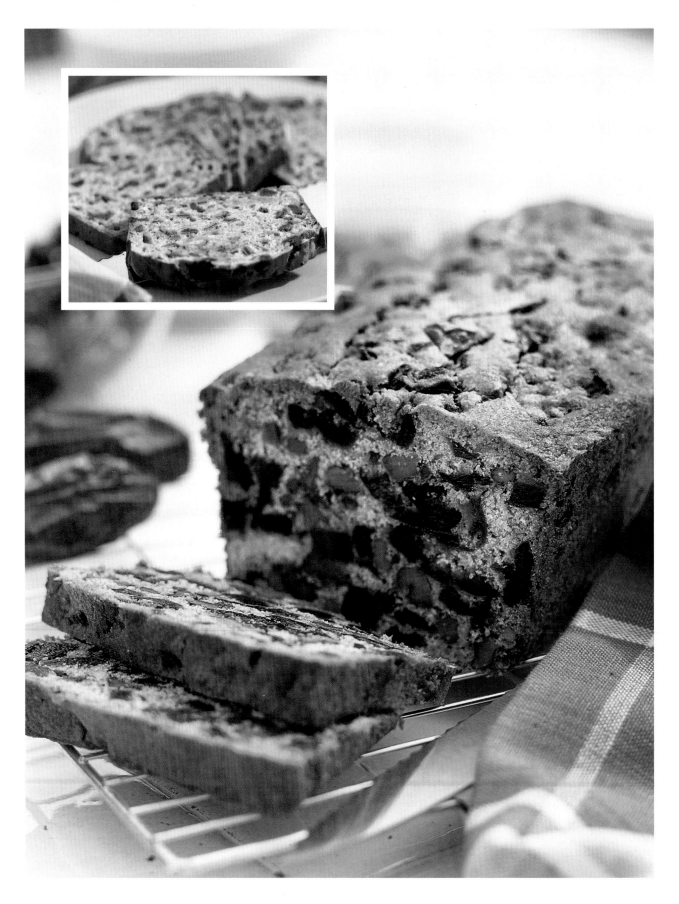

DATE & BANANA LOAF

This is a sumptuously spicy, moist fruit loaf that contains no extra fat or sugar, and relies completely on the natural sugar content of the fruits for its sweetness. Try it for yourself – it's very easy to make.

1 Preheat oven to 180°C, gas mark 4.

2 Lightly grease and line a 900 g loaf tin with non-stick baking parchment.

3 Put the chopped dates, bananas, egg and milk into a blender or food processor and process for a minute or two until the mixture is smooth.

4 Sift the flour, salt, cinnamon and ginger into a mixing bowl, then add the fruit mixture and stir until thoroughly blended.

5 Turn the mixture into the prepared tin and bake in the centre of the oven for about 30 minutes. If the loaf is fairly brown on the top, turn the heat to 160°C, gas mark 3. If not, leave it as it is, and bake for a further 25–30 minutes, or until a skewer inserted in the centre comes out clean.

6 Leave the loaf to cool in the tin for 10 minutes, then turn it out and leave it to cool completely on a wire rack.

175 g 'ready-to-eat' dried, stoned dates, coarsely chopped

3 x 175 g bananas, peeled and coarsely chopped

1 large egg

125 ml skimmed milk

225 g self-raising flour

Pinch of salt

½ teaspoon ground cinnamon

½ teaspoon ground ginger

Makes 15 slices

FRUIT & WALNUT LOAF

Walnuts add their own rich flavour and texture to this satisfyingly rich loaf, while the fruits contribute their own sweetness and moisture. It's also healthily low in sugar and high in fibre, making this an excellent choice for diabetics.

1 Preheat the oven to 180 C, gas mark 4.

2 Cream the butter and sugar together and mix in the beaten egg.

3 Mix in the self-raising and wholewheat flour and baking powder, and stir in the milk until the mixture is a thick consistency.

4 Add the fruit and nuts and mix well.

5 Spoon the mixture into a 900 g greased loaf tin and bake for 1 hour (test to ensure that it is fully cooked by inserting a skewer and checking that it comes out clean).

6 Cool the loaf on a wire rack before slicing.

85 g butter

115 g caster sugar

1 large egg, beaten

115 g self-raising flour

115 g wholewheat flour

½ teaspoon baking powder

200 ml skimmed milk

200 g fresh dates, stoned and chopped into small pieces

200 g soft dried plums, stoned and chopped into small pieces

115 g walnut pieces, roughly chopped

Makes 18–20 pieces

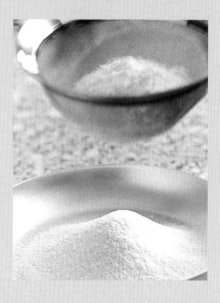

85 g fine plain flour

Pinch of salt

1 teaspoon baking powder

3 medium eggs

85 g caster sugar

1 teaspoon vanilla essence

15 g caster sugar, to dredge

55 g reduced-sugar raspberry jam, to fill

Makes 8 slices

QUICK & EASY SWISS ROLL

This feather-light confection takes just minutes to bake and is quite simple to prepare. The only tricky part is rolling it up, so follow the instructions carefully. If the edges seem a little crisp after baking, it's a good idea to trim them before rolling or the sponge may crack. Any flavour of reduced-sugar jam may be used.

1   Preheat the oven to 220°C, gas mark 7.

2   Lightly grease and line a Swiss roll tin with non-stick baking parchment.

3   Sift the flour, salt and baking powder into a bowl.

4   In another larger bowl suspended over a pan of hot water, whisk the eggs and caster sugar with an electric beater until they are thick and creamy.

5   Add the vanilla essence and lightly fold in the flour mixture, using a large metal spoon.

6   Tip the sponge mixture into the prepared tin, spreading it out evenly to the corners and bake for 6–8 minutes. Remove it from the oven when the sponge feels springy to the touch.

7   Place a sheet of baking parchment on top of a clean tea-towel and sprinkle the parchment with the dredging sugar. Turn the sponge out onto the parchment, crust side down, and remove the lining paper.

8   Make a shallow cut half-way through the sponge about 2½ cm from one of the long edges. Turn this section of sponge over to make an initial 'roll.'

9   Carefully roll up the rest of the sponge using the baking parchment.

10 Leave the roll to cool on a wire rack and when it is cold carefully unroll it and spread with the jam about 1 cm from the edges.

11 Roll it up again carefully and slice before serving.

WALNUT LAYER CAKE

*This light, low-fat mixture makes a delicate, melt-in-the-mouth cake.
It's versatile too – you can serve it for an informal tea-time treat, but it
would also be perfect for a birthday cake. You can vary the filling and
topping as the mood takes you.*

1 Preheat the oven to 160°C, gas mark 3

2 Lightly grease and line a Swiss roll tin with non-stick baking parchment.

3 Sift the flour, salt and baking powder into a bowl.

4 Cream the low-fat spread and sugar together until light and fluffy, then
   beat in the almond essence.

5 Add the beaten eggs, a little at a time, beating well after each addition.
   Add a little of the flour mixture if there is any sign of curdling.

6 Now add the remaining flour mixture, a little at a time, gently but
   thoroughly folding it in with a large metal spoon. Add the milk to give a
   smooth consistency and stir in the chopped walnuts.

7 Turn the mixture into the prepared tin, smoothing it evenly into the corners
   and bake for 25 minutes. A skewer inserted in the centre should come out
   clean. If it's at all sticky, turn the oven down to 150°C, gas mark 2 and bake
   for a further 10 minutes.

8 Cool in the tin for 15 minutes, then very gently remove from the tin, peel
   off the baking parchment and leave on a wire rack until completely cold.

9 Cut horizontally into 3 oblong sponges, to use as 3 layers, trimming the
   tops of 2 of them, if necessary, to provide flat surfaces.

10 To make the filling, mix the low-fat soft cheese and the icing sugar and
   spread over 2 of the layers.

11 Top with the 3rd layer of sponge and decorate it with icing and halved
   walnuts. (Dip the blade of a knife in hot water to give icing a smooth and
   even surface.)

RASPBERRY LAYER CAKE

Follow steps 1–9, using vanilla essence instead of almond and omitting the
walnuts. To make the filling, mix 115 g low-fat soft cheese with 55 g reduced
sugar raspberry jam and spread over 2 layers. Add the top layer, ice it as above,
and decorate with 25 g glacé cherries.

250 g self-raising flour

Pinch of salt

2 teaspoons baking powder

100 g low-fat spread, at room
temperature

100 g caster sugar

1 teaspoon almond essence

2 large eggs, beaten

125 ml semi-skimmed milk

55 g chopped walnuts

FOR THE FILLING

115 g low-fat soft cheese

25 g icing sugar

FOR THE TOPPING

40 g sieved icing sugar, mixed with
2½ teaspoons warm water

58 g halved walnuts, to decorate

Makes 12 pieces

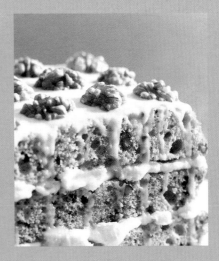

CARROT CAKE

This moist carrot cake has a delicious flavour. What's more, you can easily transform it into a passion cake by using the soft cheese as a topping and sprinkling with some chopped nuts. Or, if you prefer, simply omit the cheese altogether.

140 g wholemeal self-raising flour

Pinch of salt

1 teaspoon baking powder

1 teaspoon ground mixed spice

1 teaspoon ground ginger

55 g soft dark brown sugar

115 g sultanas, soaked overnight in 125 ml unsweetened orange juice

4 medium carrots, peeled and finely-grated

1 tablespoon sunflower oil

2 medium egg whites, at room temperature

100 g low-fat soft cheese beaten with 2 teaspoons sieved icing sugar, to fill

Makes 12 slices

1   Preheat the oven to 170°C, gas mark 3. Lightly grease a 900 g loaf tin and line it with non-stick baking parchment.

2   Sift the flour, salt, baking powder, mixed spice and ginger into a large bowl, tipping in any bran left in the sieve.

3   Stir in the sugar, sultanas with their juice, carrots and oil and mix well.

4   Beat the egg whites until they stand up in soft peaks, then fold lightly but thoroughly into the carrot mixture, using a large metal spoon.

5   Turn into the tin and bake in the centre of the oven for about 1 hour–1 ¼ hour, or until a skewer inserted in the centre of the cake comes out clean.

6   Cool in the tin for 10 minutes, then turn out onto a wire rack and peel off the baking parchment. When completely cold, cut in half horizontally and fill with the sweetened soft cheese.

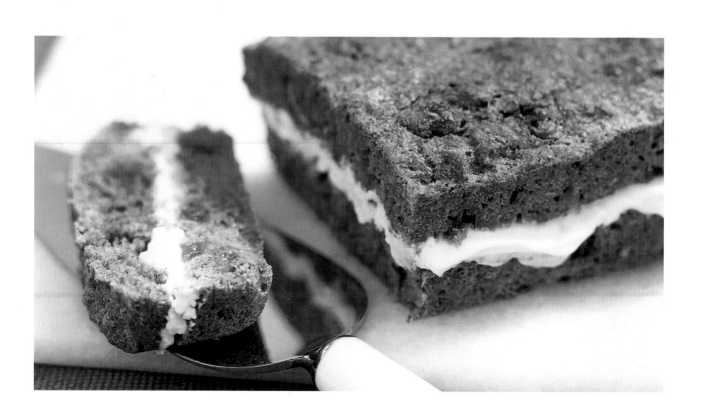

ORANGE & ALMOND CAKE

Next time you decide to make freshly-squeezed orange juice, don't throw away the fruit 'shells.' Grate the zest finely and use it in this typically Portuguese tea-time treat. Traditionally the ratio of flour and almonds is half and half, but this version gives a much lighter texture.

1 Preheat the oven to 180°C, gas mark 4.

2 Lightly-grease the base of a 20 cm non-stick sandwich tin and line with baking parchment.

3 Sift the flour, salt and baking powder together.

4 Beat the eggs until they are light and frothy.

5 Beat the spread and caster sugar together until smooth and creamy. Add the beaten eggs gradually, beating well between each addition. If the mixture shows any signs of curdling, beat in a little of the flour mixture.

6 Stir in the flour mixture together with the ground almonds, almond essence and orange zest and mix lightly to a soft dropping (but not runny) consistency, adding a little orange juice or water if necessary.

7 Turn into the prepared tin, smooth the top with a palette knife, and bake in the centre of the oven for about 45–50 minutes, or until a skewer comes out clean when inserted through the centre.

8 Strip off the baking parchment and leave the cake to cool on a wire rack.

85 g plain flour

Pinch salt

2 teaspoons baking powder

2 large eggs

85 g low-fat spread, at room temperature

85 g caster sugar

25 g ground almonds

½ teaspoon almond essence

2 teaspoons finely-grated orange zest

Makes 10 slices

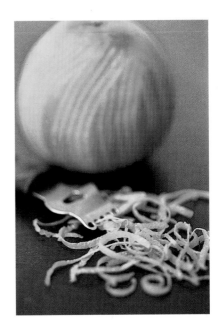

RICH FRUIT CAKE

450 g dried mixed fruit

150 ml dry cider

115 g glacé cherries, chopped

55 g chopped mixed nuts

115 g self-raising flour

115 g wholemeal self-raising flour

1 teaspoon baking powder

2 teaspoons mixed spice

115 ml sunflower oil

3 medium eggs

175 g dark muscovado sugar

2 teaspoons brandy or rum essence

Maturing time: 3 days–4 weeks

Makes 20 slices

Here's a cake that's rich, fruity and full of goodness. Because it's made with sunflower oil rather than butter, it's healthily low in saturated fat and both the fruit and nuts are packed with valuable fibre. It is ideal for icing and decorating on special occasions such as Christmas, birthdays and other anniversaries.

1   Soak the fruit overnight in the cider, then mix in the cherries and nuts.

2   Preheat the oven to 170°C, gas mark 3. Lightly grease and line a 20 cm cake tin with non-stick baking parchment.

3   Sift the 2 flours with the baking powder and mixed spice, emptying any leftover bran into the bowl.

4   In a large bowl, beat the sunflower oil with the eggs and sugar. Add the brandy or rum essence, fruit, nuts and cider and mix thoroughly.

5   Stir the dry ingredients, a bit at a time, into the egg and fruit mixture, using a large metal spoon and mixing all the time until a soft, dropping consistency is obtained.

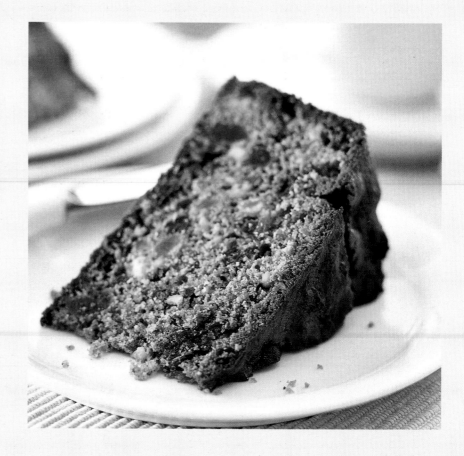

6 Stir the mixture into the prepared tin and bake for 1 hour 20 minutes or until a skewer inserted in the centre comes out clean. If the top gets too brown, cover it with a double sheet of baking parchment.

7 Allow to cool in the tin for about 1 hour, then transfer to a wire rack. When cold, store in an airtight in for at least 3 days before serving.

MINCE PIES

These mouthwatering little pies are relatively low in fat and sugar, yet they are still meltingly moist and full of festive flavour. This home-made mincemeat is fragrant with added cinnamon, brandy essence and ginger. The recipe makes 350 g of mincemeat, so there is enough for 2 batches of pies. Meanwhile, it will keep for a week in a screw-top jar in the refrigerator.

1 Soak the fruits, cinnamon, ginger, suet, orange juice, and the brandy essence overnight.

2 Sift the flour and salt into a bowl and rub in the fats lightly with your fingertips until the mixture resembles fine breadcrumbs.

3 Add the water, and very quickly mix with a fork or a palette knife until the mixture clings together, leaving the sides of the bowl clean.

4 Turn the mixture out onto a lightly floured board and knead lightly to form a soft dough (the less it is handled, the lighter the pastry will be).

5 Put the pastry into a polythene bag and chill in the fridge for 30 minutes. After 15 minutes, preheat the oven to 200°C, gas mark 6, and lightly grease a 12-hole, non-stick bun tin.

6 Roll out half of the pastry then, using a 6 cm pastry cutter, cut out 12 circles to line the prepared tin.

7 Spoon half the mincemeat (175 g) into the prepared pastry cases.

8 Dampen the edges of the pastry with a little water, then roll out the remainder of the pastry to make lids for the pies, pressing each one down gently but firmly to seal.

9 Brush the tops of the pies lightly with milk and bake for 15–20 minutes until crisp and golden.

FOR THE MINCEMEAT

175 g dried mixed fruit

140 g dessert apple, peeled, cored and sliced

1 teaspoon each powdered cinnamon and ginger

25 g reduced-fat suet

75 ml unsweetened orange juice

½ teaspoon rum or brandy essence

FOR THE PASTRY

175 g plain flour

Pinch of salt

40 g polyunsaturated margarine, diced

40 g white vegetable fat, diced

3 tablespoons ice-cold water

2 teaspoons skimmed milk, to glaze

Makes 12 pies

Peanut & White Chocolate Cookies

200 g plain flour

½ teaspoon baking powder

100 g reduced-fat spread

70 g sugar

85 g crunchy peanut butter

50 g white chocolate drops

1 egg, beaten

35 g unsalted peanuts

Makes 25 cookies

A well-stocked cookie jar is sure to be popular with everyone in the family – especially when you fill it with these crunchy treats. Commercially-made cookies often contain additives to make them last longer, so it makes sense to bake your own, so you know exactly what you're eating. These are packed with nutritious peanuts and raisins, and have a typical home-made appearance, with their uneven shapes and crumbly texture.

1 Preheat the oven to 190°C. gas mark 5.

2 In a bowl, mix together the flour and the baking powder. Cut in the reduced-fat spread with a palette knife, and rub it in lightly with your fingertips until the mixture resembles fine breadcrumbs.

3 Stir in the sugar, peanut butter and chocolate and mix well.

4 Mix in the egg to make a firm dough (you will find it easier to use your hands as the mixture gets firmer).

5 Form the dough into 25 equal-size balls and press them onto a lightly floured baking tray. Press down each one with the back of a fork to make a pattern and to give each cookie an uneven texture.

6 Decorate the top with the peanuts and bake for 10–12 minutes until golden brown. Cool on a wire rack.

FRUIT & NUT COOKIES

For a lower fat alternative, you could use chopped apricots or sultanas as a substitute for the chocolate.

LOW-SUGAR SHORTBREAD

Though it is considerably lower in sugar and fat than most shortbreads, this still has a delicious buttery flavour. The ground rice gives it a satisfyingly crunchy texture.

1 Preheat the oven to 150°C, gas mark 2.

2 Lightly grease a 20 cm round sandwich tin and line it with non-stick baking parchment.

3 Cream the butter until it is light and fluffy, then beat in the caster sugar.

4 Add the sifted flour and ground rice, a little at a time, and mix lightly each time. Shape the dough into a circle to fit the prepared tin.

5 Crimp the edges with the handle of a fork, cut into 8 wedges and bake in the centre of the oven for about 50 minutes until golden.

6 Remove the lining paper, dredge with sugar and cool on a wire rack.

85 g butter

35 g caster sugar

85 g plain white flour

85 g ground rice

15 g caster sugar, to decorate

Makes 8 pieces

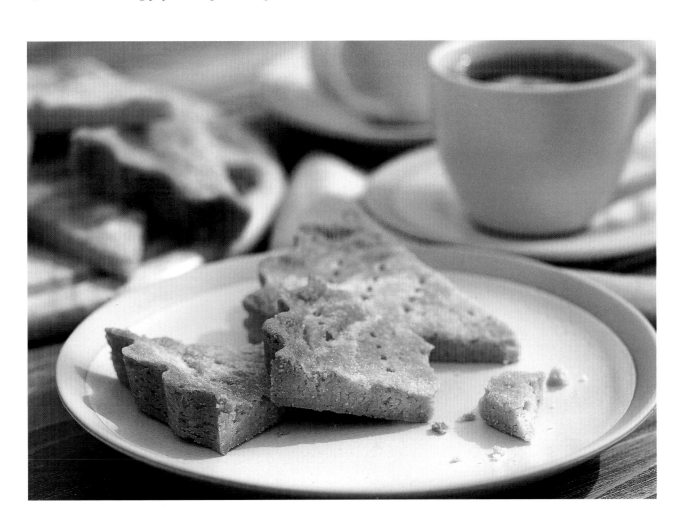

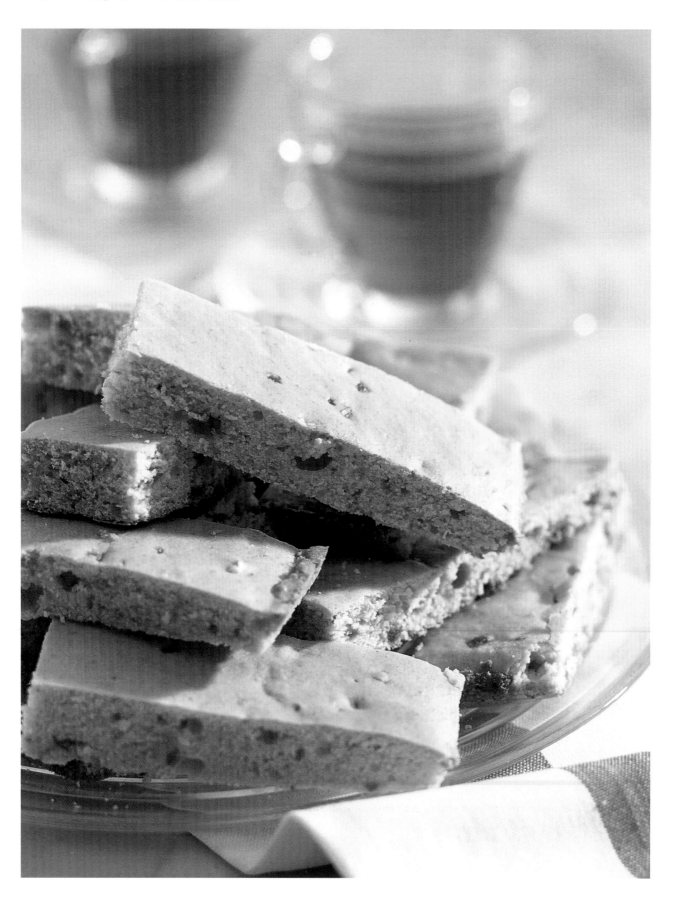

CHERRY ALMOND FINGERS

You'll certainly enjoy the aromas of almonds and cherries while these delicious home-made fingers are baking in the oven. They're easy to cook and even easier to eat, making this a perfect tea-time treat.

1 Preheat the oven to 160°C, gas mark 3. Lightly grease and line a Swiss roll tin with non-stick baking parchment.

2 Sift the flour and baking powder. In a large bowl, cream the spread and sugar until light and fluffy. Stir in the ground almonds and cherries.

3 Mix the beaten egg with the milk and almond essence, and gradually beat into the creamed fat and sugar, adding a little of the flour mixture if there is any sign of curdling.

4 Beat in the rest of the flour mixture, turn into the prepared tin and bake for about 35 minutes or until a skewer inserted in the centre comes out clean.

5 Remove the baking parchment, allow to cool on a wire rack and when completely cold, cut into fingers before serving.

225 g plain flour

2 teaspoons baking powder

115 g low-fat spread

25 g caster sugar

55 g ground almonds

85 g glacé cherries, finely chopped

1 large egg, beaten

175 ml skimmed milk

1 teaspoon almond essence

Makes 16 fingers

FRUITY FLAPJACKS

These flapjacks are crammed with fruit and make great between-meal snacks, as they also contain oats to stabilize your blood sugar. Any mixture of fruit can be used – try dried plums or raisins, or add some sesame or sunflower seeds for a different flavour and texture.

1 Preheat the oven to 180°C, gas mark 4.

2 Mix the oats, dried fruit and cinnamon together in a large bowl.

3 Place the butter and sugar in a saucepan, and stir over a low heat until the sugar is melted.

4 Add to the oat mixture and stir thoroughly until it is well combined.

5 Press the mixture into a non-stick baking tray (about 18 cm square).

6 Bake for about 25 minutes until lightly browned.

7 Leave to cool in the tray and cut into fingers when still slightly warm.

175 g rolled oats

70 g dried apricots, chopped

55 g dried pineapple, chopped

25 g dried banana chips, chopped

70 g dried mango, chopped

55 g dried cranberries

½ teaspoon ground cinnamon

125 g butter

100 g soft brown sugar

Makes 25 flapjacks

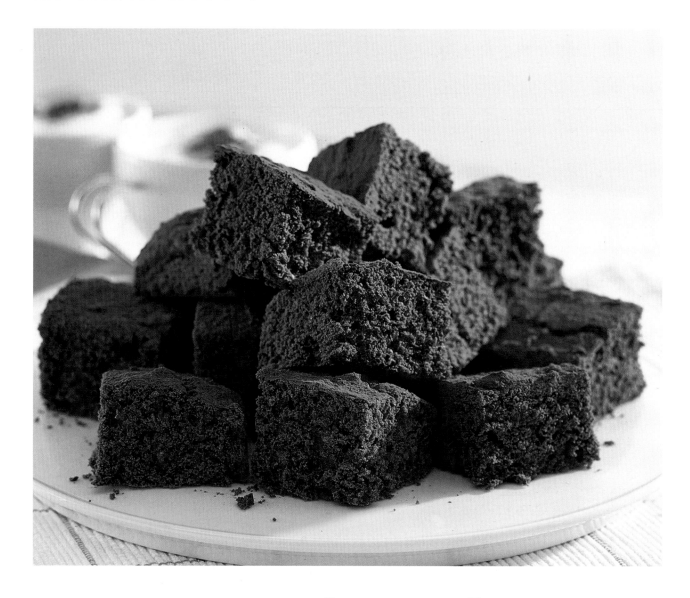

CHOCOLATE BROWNIES

225 g wholemeal self-raising flour

Pinch of salt

1 teaspoon baking powder

25 g dark cocoa powder

150 g reduced-fat spread

55 g caster sugar

2 medium eggs, beaten

100 ml skimmed milk

Makes 16 brownies

These deliciously dark, moist, chocolate-flavoured treats are perfect just as they are, and they certainly don't need the traditional coating of sugary icing.

1 Preheat the oven to 180°C, gas mark 4.

2 Lightly grease a 20 cm square cake tin and line the base with non-stick baking parchment.

3 Sift the flour, salt, baking powder and cocoa powder into a large bowl, tipping in any leftover bran in the sieve.

4 Cream the reduced-fat spread and sugar together until light and fluffy.

5 Beat in the eggs, a little at a time, adding a little of the flour mixture if there is any sign of curdling.

6 Add the rest of the flour and mix it in thoroughly.

7 Finally, beat in the milk, spoon the mixture into the prepared cake tin and bake for 25 minutes. Then, turn the gas down to 150°C, gas mark 2, and bake for a further 15–20 minutes, or until a skewer inserted in the centre comes out clean.

8 Cool in the tin for 15 minutes, peel off the lining paper and leave to cool completely on a wire rack.

9 Cut into 16 squares and dust with cocoa powder before serving.

EASY IRISH SODA BREAD

This recipe is based on a traditional Irish soda bread. If you can't get buttermilk, use semi-skimmed milk instead. Because bicarbonate of soda is used as the raising agent, it will start to 'work' very quickly when it mixes with the milk, so make sure that you have your oven heated and the baking sheet(s) greased before you start.

350 g wholemeal flour
115 g unbleached white flour
½ teaspoon salt
1 teaspoon bicarbonate of soda
15 g polyunsaturated margarine
300 ml buttermilk
Serves 12 (makes 2 loaves, each serving 6)

1 Preheat the oven to 230°C, gas mark 8 and lightly grease 1 large (or 2 medium-sized) baking sheets.

2 Sift both the flours with the salt and bicarbonate of soda into a large bowl. Set aside any bran remaining in the sieve.

3 Lightly rub in the margarine, add the buttermilk and mix quickly to a soft but manageable dough. If it's too dry to handle, add a little water.

4 Knead on a lightly-floured board for 1 minute or so, then cut in half and shape into 2 rounds.

5 Roll out the rounds to about 2½ cm thickness, and place them onto the greased baking sheet(s).

6 Score each round quite deeply to make 6 wedges in each. Sprinkle lightly with the reserved bran and bake the loaves for about 25 minutes, or until risen and golden.

7 Cool on a wire rack.

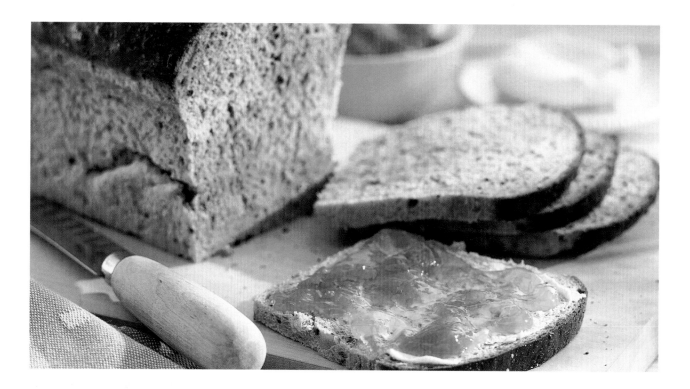

FARMHOUSE GRANARY BREAD

500 g granary flour

Pinch of salt

½ x 7g sachet easy-blend dried yeast

25 ml sunflower oil

300 ml warm water

1 small egg white, lightly-beaten (optional)

Makes a 900 g loaf (15 slices)

It's very satisfying to make your own bread, and this granary loaf has a wonderfully evocative aroma while it's baking. A small egg white is used to glaze the top, but this is optional – it does, however, give a more attractive glossy appearance. Serve the bread warm or cold, but for best results bring it to the table when it's still warm, and watch how quickly it disappears.

1   Put the flour and salt into a large bowl, then add the yeast and mix well.

2   Add the oil and water and mix thoroughly to make a pliable dough (if it is too dry to handle easily, add a little extra water.)

3   Knead the dough for about 6–8 minutes, or until it is smooth and elastic.

4   Shape the dough to fit a 900 g lightly-oiled loaf tin, lined with non-stick baking parchment. Cover it with a clean tea-towel and leave in a warm place for about 1 hour or until it is doubled in size.

5   Preheat the oven to 230°C, gas mark 8.

6   Brush the top of the bread with lightly-beaten egg white and bake for 30–35 minutes until it is golden.

7   Turn out and cool on a wire rack. Serve with low-fat spread and reduced-sugar jam, if desired.

Nutritional Analysis

The nutritional information for each recipe refers to a single serving, unless otherwise stated. Optional ingredients are not included. The figures are intended as a guide only. If salt is given in a measured amount in the recipe it has been included in the analysis; if the recipe suggests adding a pinch of salt or seasoning to taste, salt has not been included.

p.12 Oat Cookies with Raisins & Sour Cherries
116–100 cals; 2–1.5g protein; 5–4g fat; 2.5–2.0g saturated fat; 18–15g carbohydrate; 0.7–0.6g fibre; 490–410 Kjoules; 21–17 mg cholesterol; 64–54 mg sodium

p.12 Home-made Crunchy Muesli
190 cals 5 g protein; 7 g fat; 0.5 g saturated fat; 29 g carbohydrate; 2.5 g fibre; 802 Kjoules; 0 mg cholesterol; 16 mg sodium

p.13 Apricot Bran Breakfast Muffins
156cals; 4.5g protein; 6g fat; 1g saturated fat; 22g carbohydrate; 4g fibre; 657 Kjoules; 32 mg cholesterol; 147mg sodium

p.14 Fruity Breakfast Pancakes
132 cals; 3g protein; 7g fat; 1.5g saturated fat; 15g carbohydrate; 1g fibre; 553 Kjoules; 30mg cholesterol; 97mg sodium

p.15 Honey Grilled Grapefruit with Toasted Sesame Seeds
81cals; 1.5g protein; 2g fat; 0.3g saturated fat; 14.5g carbohydrate; 1.5g fibre; 342 Kjoules; 0 mg cholesterol; 5 mg sodium

p.15 Banana & Mango Yogurt Smoothie with Wheatgerm
250cals; 12g protein; 2.5g fat; 1g saturated fat; 49g carbohydrate; 4.5g fibre; 1069 Kjoules; 6mg cholesterol; 128mg sodium

p.16 Scrambled Eggs with Smoked Salmon
150cals; 15g protein; 9g fat; 2g saturated fat; 2g carbohydrate; 0.5g fibre; 616Kjoules 245mg cholesterol; 725mg sodium

p.16 Eggs Florentine
219cals; 13g protein; 12g fat; 5g saturated fat; 13g carbohydrate; 3g fibre; 916Kjoules 248mg cholesterol; 390mg sodium

p.17 Salmon Kedgeree with Fresh Coriander
445cals; 24g protein; 17g fat; 3g saturated fat; 42g carbohydrate; 0.7g fibre; 1857 Kjoules; 161mg cholesterol; 235mg sodium

p.19 Smoked Haddock Souffle Omelette with Croutons
450cals; 35g protein; 29g fat; 8g saturated fat; 14.5g carbohydrate; 2g fibre; 1889 Kjoules; 417mg cholesterol; 1444 mg sodium

p.20 Wild Mushroom Toasts
291cals; 10g protein; 9g fat; 2g saturated fat; 46g carbohydrate; 5g fibre; 1233Kjoules; 0mg cholesterol; 261mg sodium

p.21 Potato Cakes
50cals; 1g protein; 1g fat; 0.5g saturated fat; 9.5g carbohydrate; 0.7g fibre; 228 Kjoules; 3mg cholesterol; 44 mg sodium

p.24 Prawn & Apple Pitta Pockets
260cals; 16g protein; 4g fat; 0.2g saturated fat; 43g carbohydrate; 2g fibre; 1087Kjoules; 39mg cholesterol; 1088mg sodium

p.24 Layered Mediterranean Sandwich
220cals; 12g protein; 8g fat; 4g saturated fat; 28g carbohydrate; 2g fibre; 929Kjoules; 19mg cholesterol; 522mg sodium

p.25 Goat's Cheese, Tomato & Ciabatta Grill
200cals; 8g protein; 7g fat; 3g saturated fat; 26g carbohydrate; 1g fibre; 830Kjoules; 0mg cholesterol; 400mg sodium

p.26 Portuguese Sardine Salad
630cals; 56g protein; 31g fat; 8g saturated fat; 34g carbohydrate; 3.5g fibre; 2630Kjoules; 0mg cholesterol; 611mg sodium

p.26 Tuna & Dill Salad with Fresh Vegetable Crudite
130cals; 15g protein; 1g fat; 0.4g saturated fat; 16g carbohydrate; 3g fibre; 552Kjoules; 27mg cholesterol; 397mg sodium

p.27 Avocado with Warm Shredded Chicken & Walnut Salad
560cals; 28g protein; 47g fat; 9g saturated fat; 6g carbohydrate; 6g fibre; 2335Kjoules; 64mg cholesterol; 175mg sodium

p.28 Warm Lentils & Chilli Beans with Smoked Bacon
380cals; 29g protein; 11g fat; 4g saturated fat; 42g carbohydrate; 10g fibre; 1589Kjoules; 32mg cholesterol; 827mg sodium

p.28 Bean & Vegetable Stew
237cals; 10g protein; 4g fat; 1g saturated fat; 42g carbohydrate; 11g fibre; 1004Kjoules; 0mg cholesterol; 431mg sodium

p.29 Tuscan Bread Salad with Red Onion & Mozzarella
360cals; 17g protein; 19g fat; 7g saturated fat; 33g carbohydrate; 3g fibre; 28Kjoules; 546mg cholesterol; 1520mg sodium

p.29 Savoury Popcorn Snack
27cals; 0.5g protein; 1g fat; 0g saturated fat; 4g carbohydrate; 0g fibre; 110Kjoules; 0mg cholesterol; 0mg sodium

p.31 Potato, Red Pepper & Onion Frittata
170cals; 9g protein; 10g fat; 2.5g saturated fat; 12g carbohydrate; 1.5g fibre; 716Kjoules; 241mg cholesterol; 95mg sodium

p.31 Vegetable Gratin
260cals; 15g protein; 14g fat; 7g saturated fat; 20g carbohydrate; 6g fibre; 1082Kjoules; 32mg cholesterol; 420mg sodium

p. 32 Pizza with Three-coloured Peppers & Beans
470cals; 22g protein; 12g fat; 5g saturated fat; 70g carbohydrate; 12g fibre; 1971Kjoules; 19mg cholesterol; 697mg sodium

p.34 Filled Jacket Potatoes – with Avocado & Prawns
315cals; 11g protein; 13g fat; 3g saturated fat; 40g carbohydrate; 4g fibre; 1321Kjoules; 20mg cholesterol; 416mg sodium

– with Tuna Tricolor
263cals; 12g protein; 6g fat; 0.5g saturated fat; 43g carbohydrate; 3.5g fibre; 1111Kjoules; 16mg cholesterol; 179mg sodium

– with Pesto and Smoked Ham
344cals; 14g protein; 16g fat; 4g saturated fat; 40g carbohydrate; 3g fibre; 1440Kjoules; 27mg cholesterol; 437mg sodium

p.35 Baked Cheesy Triangles
268cals; 18g protein; 8g fat; 4g saturated fat; 33g carbohydrate; 4g fibre; 1134Kjoules; 72mg cholesterol; 627mg sodium

p.35 Stuffed Peppers
236cals; 9g protein; 4g fat; 1g saturated fat 41g carbohydrate; 4g fibre; 987Kjoules; 3mg cholesterol; 57mg sodium

p.38 Pumpkin Soup with Roast Parsnip Crisps
120–80 cals; 5–3.5 g protein; 4.5–3g fat; 1–0.6g saturated fat; 16–10.5g carbohydrate; 4.5–3g fibre; 503–335 Kjoules; 2–1 mg cholesterol; 218–145mg sodium

p.39 Bean & Pasta Soup with Basil
280–190cals; 8–5g protein; 10–7g fat; 3–2g saturated fat; 25–16g carbohydrate; 5.5–4g fibre; 1177–785 Kjoules; 0 mg cholesterol; 292–134mg sodium

p.40 Red Lentil Soup
228–152cals; 14–10g protein; 1–0.8g fat; 0.2–0.1g saturated fat; 42–28g carbohydrate; 6–4g fibre; 966–644Kjoules; 0mg cholesterol; 150–100mg sodium

p.40 Spinach & Onion Soup
90cals; 3g protein; 3g fat; 0.5g saturated fat; 5g carbohydrate; 2g fibre; 374Kjoules; 0mg cholesterol; 288mg sodium

p.41 Fish & Potato Soup
242–162cals; 28–19g protein; 3–2g fat; 1–0.8g saturated fat; 29–19g carbohydrate; 4–3g fibre; 1028–685Kjoules; 48–32mg cholesterol; 1020–680mg sodium

p.41 Garlic Bread
190cals; 5g protein; 7g fat; 2g saturated fat; 28g carbohydrate; 0.8g fibre; 795Kjoules; 1mg cholesterol; 374 mg sodium

p.43 Garlic Prawns
70cals; 10g protein; 3g fat; 0.4g saturated fat; 0g carbohydrate; 0g fibre; 282Kjoules; 110mg cholesterol; 107mg sodium

p.43 Monkfish Kebabs with Lemon & Thyme
132cals; 25g protein; 3.5g fat; 0.5g saturated fat; 0g carbohydrate; 0g fibre; 560Kjoules; 23mg cholesterol; 29mg sodium

p.44 Honey-glazed Chicken Wings
277cals; 34g protein; 14g fat; 5g saturated fat; 2g carbohydrate; 0g fibre; 1157Kjoules 121mg cholesterol; 164mg sodium

p.44 Sautéed Chicken Liver with Fennel
110cals; 12g protein; 5g fat; 1g saturated fat; 4g carbohydrate; 1.5g fibre; 457Kjoules 214mg cholesterol; 54mg sodium

p.45 Mini Kebabs with Yogurt Dip
143cals; 17g protein; 7g fat; 3g saturated fat; 3g carbohydrate; 0g fibre; 598Kjoules; 61mg cholesterol; 194mg sodium

p.46 Falafels with Mint Dip
50cals; 3g protein; 1.5g fat; 0.2g saturated fat; 7g carbohydrate; 1.3g fibre; 213Kjoules; 1mg cholesterol; 145mg sodium

p.46 Roasted Baby Tomatoes & Aubergines
23cals; 1g protein; 0.5g fat; 0.1g saturated fat; 4g carbohydrate; 2g fibre; 97Kjoules; 0mg cholesterol; 9mg sodium

p.47 Crispy Potato Wedges with Cream & Chive Dip
256cals; 7g protein; 12g fat; 4.5g saturated fat; 31g carbohydrate; 2g fibre; 1075Kjoules; 0mg cholesterol; 43mg sodium

p.50 Tiger Prawn Risotto
400cals; 30g protein; 6g fat; 2.5g saturated fat; 56g carbohydrate; 3g fibre; 1686Kjoules; 205mg cholesterol; 661mg sodium

p.51 Stir-fried Squid with Lemon Grass & Ginger
380cals; 27g protein; 10g fat; 2g saturated fat; 50g carbohydrate; 5g fibre; 1624Kjoules; 270mg cholesterol; 403mg sodium

p.51 Smoked Fish Parcels
180cals; 29g protein; 2g fat; 0.2g saturated fat; 9g carbohydrate; 1.5g fibre; 760Kjoules 69mg cholesterol; 1764mg sodium

p.52 Pan-fried Cod with Pesto
490cals; 43g protein; 34g fat; 5g saturated fat; 1.5g carbohydrate; 0.5g fibre; 2018Kjoules; 100mg cholesterol; 203mg sodium

p.52 Balsamic Salmon Steaks
350cals; 33g protein; 24g fat; 4g saturated fat; 0.8g carbohydrate; 0g fibre; 1462Kjoules; 88mg cholesterol; 643mg sodium

p.53 Grilled Halibut with Red Pepper Sauce
250cals; 32g protein; 9g fat; 1g saturated fat; 9g carbohydrate; 2g fibre; 1043K joules; 88mg cholesterol; 171mg sodium

p.54 Fettuccine with Salmon, Asparagus & Lemon
540cals; 37g protein; 21g fat; 6.5g saturated fat; 50g carbohydrate; 2.5g fibre; 2282Kjoules; 57mg cholesterol; 133mg sodium

p.56 Coriander Chicken with Orange
360cals; 35g protein; 17g fat; 3g saturated fat; 17g carbohydrate; 2g fibre; 1500Kjoules; 86mg cholesterol; 311mg sodium

p.56 Chicken Breasts with Salsa
225cals; 17g protein; 16g fat; 3.5g saturated fat; 4g carbohydrate; 2g fibre; 952Kjoules; 43mg cholesterol' 118mg sodium

p.57 Chicken with Ginger
275cals; 36g protein; 10g fat; 3g saturated fat; 9g carbohydrate; 0g fibre; 1156Kjoules; 100mg cholesterol; 574mg sodium

p.58 Chicken with Cardamom
331cals; 25g protein; 15g fat; 2g saturated fat; 25g carbohydrate; 2.5g fibre; 1387Kjoules; 46mg cholesterol; 316mg sodium

p.58 Turkey with Red Onion & Watercress Salad
260cals; 38g protein; 9g fat; 2g saturated fat; 6g carbohydrate; 0.5g fibre; 1084Kjoules; 104mg cholesterol; 92mg sodium

p.60 Turkey Fricassee with Olive Oil Mash
430cals; 47g protein; 12g fat; 3gsaturated fat; 34g carbohydrate; 4g fibre; 1812Kjoules; 84mg cholesterol; 322mg sodium

p.61 Duck Breasts with Coconut
180cals; 17g protein; 10g fat; 7g saturated fat; 4g carbohydrate; 1.5g fibre; 766Kjoules; 83mg cholesterol; 128mg sodium

p.61 Sweet & Sour Duck
324cals; 26g protein; 8g fat; 2g saturated fat; 39g carbohydrate; 3g fibre; 1370Kjoules; 127mg cholesterol; 801mg sodium

p.62 Smoked Sausage Cassoulet
400cals; 25g protein; 17g fat; 2.5g saturated fat; 38g carbohydrate; 11g fibre; 1676Kjoules; 44mg cholesterol; 1786mg sodium

p.62 Italian Meatballs
550cals; 39g protein; 10g fat; 3g saturated fat; 76g carbohydrate; 4g fibre; 2331Kjoules; 69mg cholesterol; 296mg sodium

p.64 Beef with Green Pepper & Noodles
570cals; 38g protein; 18g fat; 5g saturated fat; 67g carbohydrate; 4g fibre; 2393Kjoules; 93mg cholesterol; 876mg sodium

p.64 Griddled Fillet Steak with Field Mushrooms
275cals; 27g protein; 14g fat; 8g saturated fat; 10g carbohydrate; 2g fibre; 1146Kjoules; 84mg cholesterol; 251mg sodium

p.65 Lamb with Apricots
290cals; 23g protein; 10g fat; 4g saturated fat; 22g carbohydrate; 3g fibre; 1233 Kjoules; 79mg cholesterol; 331mg sodium

p.66 Lamb Baked in Yogurt
380cals; 41g protein; 20g fat; 8g saturated fat; 8g carbohydrate; 1g fibre; 1586Kjoules; 135mg cholesterol; 541mg sodium

p.66 Venison in Red Wine
400cals; 38g protein; 22g fat; 3g saturated fat; 5g carbohydrate; 2g fibre; 1665Kjoules; 75mg cholesterol; 274mg sodium

p.67 Broccoli & Herb Pasta
376cals; 18g protein; 7g fat; 2g saturated fat; 64g carbohydrate; 6g fibre; 1593Kjoules; 6mg cholesterol; 125mg sodium

p.67 Vegetable Pilaf
290cals; 12g protein; 2.5g fat; 0.3g saturated fat; 55g carbohydrate; 5g fibre; 1222Kjoules; 0mg cholesterol; 592mg sodium

p.68 Polenta with Tomatoes, Porcini & Goat's Cheese
390cals; 11g protein; 16g fat; 4g saturated fat; 50g carbohydrate; 1.4g fibre; 1630Kjoules; 0mg cholesterol; 263mg sodium

p.69 Polenta Bruschettas with Mediterranean Vegetables
255cals; 9g protein; 9g fat; 2g saturated fat; 33g carbohydrate; 4g fibre; 1062Kjoules; 6mg cholesterol; 111mg sodium

p.69 Mixed Pepper Couscous
214cals; 5g protein; 6g fat; 1g saturated fat; 36g carbohydrate; 1.5g fibre; 892Kjoules; 0mg cholesterol; 9mg sodium

p.70 Spicy Chickpeas in Wholemeal Wraps
558cals; 22g protein; 14g fat; 2g saturated fat; 90g carbohydrate; 14g fibre; 2357Kjoules; 1mg cholesterol; 326mg sodium

p.72 Pancakes Stuffed with Spinach & Ricotta
280cals; 19g protein; 10g fat; 4g saturated fat; 29g carbohydrate; 6g fibre; 1162Kjoules; 26mg cholesterol; 328mg sodium

p.73 Penne with Roasted Vegetables
354cals; 10g protein; 10g fat; 1.5g saturated fat; 58g carbohydrate; 5g fibre; 1493Kjoules; 0mg cholesterol; 19mg sodium

p.73 Saffron Rice with Vegetables & Soft Cheese
369cals; 13g protein; 7g fat; 3g saturated fat; 58g carbohydrate; 5g fibre; 1649Kjoules; 0mg cholesterol; 397mg sodium

p.76 Lemon & Onion Roasted Potatoes
180cals; 4g protein; 6g fat; 0.1g saturated fat; 29g carbohydrate; 2.5g fibre; 755Kjoules; 0mg cholesterol; 12mg sodium

p.76 Roasted New Potatoes with Tomatoes & Herbs
112cals; 2g protein; 3g fat; 0.5g saturated fat; 20g carbohydrate; 1.5g fibre; 473Kjoules; 0mg cholesterol; 17mg sodium

p.78 Baked Sweet Potatoes with Chilli Butter
250cals; 3g protein; 5g fat; 3g saturated fat; 53g carbohydrate; 6g fibre; 1082Kjoules; 12mg cholesterol; 138mg sodium

p.78 Parsnip Croquettes
41cals; 1.5g protein; 6g fat; 1g saturated fat; 8g carbohydrate; 1g fibre; 175Kjoules; 12mg cholesterol; 28mg sodium

p.79 Sweetcorn Frites
60cals; 2g protein; 1g fat; 0.2g saturated fat; 11g carbohydrate; 0.5g fibre; 247Kjoules; 16mg cholesterol; 95mg sodium

p.79 Stir-fried Baby Corn & Mangetout
100cals; 6g protein; 6g fat; 0.6g saturated fat; 6g carbohydrate; 3g fibre; 415Kjoules; 0mg cholesterol; 33mg sodium

p.81 Roasted Mediterranean Vegetables with Pine Nuts
325cals; 9g protein; 23g fat; 2g saturated fat; 20g carbohydrate; 5g fibre; 1344Kjoules; 0mg cholesterol; 10mg sodium

p.81 Baked Tomato & Olive Salad
70cals; 1.5g protein; 4g fat; 1g saturated fat; 7g carbohydrate; 2g fibre; 293Kjoules; 0mg cholesterol; 21mg sodium

p.82 Tabouleh
180cals; 4.5g protein; 7g fat; 1g saturated fat; 26g carbohydrate; 3g fibre; 755Kjoules; 0mg cholesterol; 24mg sodium

p.83 Peppery Bean Salad
204cals; 11g protein; 7g fat; 1g saturated fat; 26g carbohydrate; 8g fibre; 863Kjoules; 4mg cholesterol; 432mg sodium

p.83 Cabbage with Caraway Seeds
55cals; 3g protein; 4g fat; 0.5g saturated fat; 5g carbohydrate; 3g fibre; 226Kjoules; 0mg cholesterol; 7mg sodium

p.83 Red Cabbage Coleslaw
131cals; 1.6g protein; 9g fat; 0g saturated fat; 12.5g carbohydrate; 4g fibre; 543Kjoules; 0mg cholesterol; 300mg sodium

p.86 Raspberry Souffle Omelette
182cals; 8g protein; 10g fat; 2g saturated fat; 17g carbohydrate; 1g fibre; 774Kjoules 235mg cholesterol; 88mg sodium

p.86 Baked Bananas with Orange
100cals; 1.5g protein; 0.3g fat; 0g saturated fat; 24g carbohydrate; 1g fibre; 414 Kjoules; 0mg cholesterol; 2mg sodium

p.87 Charred Fruit Kebabs
80cals; 1g protein; 0.5g fat; 0g saturated fat; 19g carbohydrate; 2.5g fibre; 335Kjoules; 0mg cholesterol; 4mg sodium

p.88 Amaretto & Almond Stuffed Peaches
190cals; 3g protein; 10g fat; 5g saturated fat; 17g carbohydrate; 2g fibre; 811Kjoules; 9mg cholesterol; 31mg sodium

p.88 Poached Pears with
Raspberry Coulis
75cals; 1g protein; 0.3g fat; 0.1g
saturated fat; 17g carbohydrate; 5g
fibre; 315Kjoules; 0mg cholesterol; 6mg
sodium

p.90 Wholesome Bread & Butter Pudding
273cals; 13g protein; 10g fat; 4.5g saturated fat; 35g carbohydrate; 2.3g fibre;
1149Kjoules; 178mg cholesterol; 366mg
sodium

p.90 Apple & Plum Crumble
310cals; 7g protein; 5g fat; 1g saturated
fat; 62g carbohydrate; 6g fibre;
1311Kjoules; 3mg cholesterol; 45mg
sodium

p.91 Black Forest Crepes
275cals; 8.5g protein; 10g fat; 4.5g
saturated fat; 40g carbohydrate; 1g fibre;
1161Kjoules; 61mg cholesterol; 166mg
sodium

p.92 Apricot & Apple Tarte Tatin
226cals; 4g protein; 4g fat; 1.4g
saturated fat; 45g carbohydrate; 4g
fibre; 959Kjoules; 3mg cholesterol; 106mg
sodium

p.93 Chilled Lemon & Lime Mousse
328cals; 5g protein; 21g fat; 13g saturated
fat; 29g carbohydrate; 0g fibre;
1371Kjoules; 58mg cholesterol; 18mg sodium

p.95 Chocolate & Almond Custard Tart
251cals; 7g protein; 14g fat; 3g saturated
fat; 25g carbohydrate; 1.5g fibre;
1050Kjoules; 80mg cholesterol; 189mg
sodium

p.96 Lemon & Sultana Cheesecake with
Cherries
250cals; 7g protein; 11g fat; 4g saturated
fat; 31g carbohydrate; 1g fibre;
1046Kjoules; 17mg cholesterol; 218mg
sodium

p.96 Petits Coeurs a la Creme
135cals; 6g protein; 5g fat; 3g
saturated fat 18g carbohydrate; 1.5g
fibre; 570Kjoules; 17mg cholesterol;
37mg sodium

p.99 Raspberry & Blueberry Shortcake
Stacks
385cals; 5g protein; 20g fat; 5g saturated
fat; 47g carbohydrate; 2g fibre;
1611Kjoules; 1mg cholesterol; 173mg
sodium

p.100 Raspberry & Ginger Sundaes
376cals; 6g protein; 21g fat; 8g saturated
fat; 41g carbohydrate; 2.5g fibre;
1580Kjoules; 6mg cholesterol; 217mg
sodium

p.100 Exotic Fruit Salad with Cardamom
160–120cals; 1.6–1.2g protein; 0.4–0.3g fat;
0g saturated fat; 40–30g carbohydrate;
5–3.5g fibre; 681–511Kjoules; 0mg cholesterol; 12–9mg sodium

p.102 Banana Ice Cream with Chocolate
& Hazelnut Topping
468cals; 13g protein; 26g fat; 12g saturated
fat; 47g carbohydrate; 1.6g fibre;
1955Kjoules; 39mg cholesterol; 208mg
sodium

p.103 Summer Berry Frozen Dessert
110cals; 4g protein; 0.6g fat; 0.3g saturated
fat; 24g carbohydrate; 2g fibre; 464Kjoules;
2mg cholesterol; 50mg sodium

p.103 Strawberry & Mascarpone Sorbet
250cals; 3g protein; 16g fat; 10g saturated
fat; 24g carbohydrate; 1g fibre;
1056Kjoules; 27mg cholesterol; 101mg
sodium

p.106 Fruit Scones
113cals; 3g protein; 3g fat; 0.6g saturated
fat; 20g carbohydrate; 1.3g fibre;
479Kjoules; 0.5mg cholesterol; 166mg
sodium

p.107 Grandma's Home-made
Gingerbread
171cals; 3g protein; 5.6g fat; 1g saturated
fat; 29g carbohydrate; 0.75g fibre;
722Kjoules; 15mg cholesterol; 190mg
sodium

p.109 Date & Banana Loaf
123cals; 3g protein; 0.7g fat; 0.2g saturated
fat; 29g carbohydrate; 1.3g fibre;
523Kjoules; 16mg cholesterol; 91mg
sodium

p.109 Fruit & Walnut Loaf
183cals; 3.6g protein; 8.8g fat; 3g saturated
fat; 24g carbohydrate; 1.8g fibre;
769Kjoules; 24mg cholesterol; 88mg
sodium

p.110 Quick & Easy Swiss Roll
129cals; 3.9g protein; 2.6g fat; 0.8g
saturated fat; 24g carbohydrate; 0.4g fibre;
544Kjoules; 88mg cholesterol; 156mg
sodium

p.111 Walnut Layer Cake
310cals; 7g protein; 15g fat; 4 saturated fat
38g carbohydrate; 1g fibre; 1300Kjoules;
40mg cholesterol; 328mg sodium

p.112 Carrot Cake
119cals; 3g protein; 2g fat; 1g saturated fat;
22g carbohydrate; 1.7g fibre; 502Kjoules;
0mg cholesterol; 99mg sodium

p.113 Orange & Almond Cake
131cals; 3.4g protein; 6.2g fat; 1.4g
saturated fat; 16g carbohydrate; 0.5g fibre;
547Kjoules; 48mg cholesterol; 230mg
sodium

p.114 Rich Fruit Cake
217cals; 3.8g protein; 5.2g fat; 1g saturated
fat; 36g carbohydrate; 1.7g fibre;
914Kjoules; 35mg cholesterol; 67mg
sodium

p.114 Mince Pies
162cals; 1.8g protein; 7.4g fat; 2.5g
saturated fat; 24g carbohydrate; 0.9g fibre;
682Kjoules; 3.2mg cholesterol; 66mg
sodium

p.116 Peanut & White Chocolate Cookies
97cals; 2.6g protein; 5g fat; 1.7g saturated
fat; 11g carbohydrate; 0.5g fibre;
408Kjoules; 11mg cholesterol; 50mg
sodium

p.117 Low Sugar Shortbread
241cals; 2.6g protein; 12g fat; 7.8g saturated fat; 32g carbohydrate; 0.6g fibre;
1012Kjoules; 33mg cholesterol; 109mg
sodium

p.119 Cherry Almond Fingers
128cals; 3.4g protein; 5.4g fat; 1g saturated
fat; 17g carbohydrate; 0.8g fibre;
532Kjoules; 15mg cholesterol; 134mg
sodium

p.119 Fruity Flapjacks
110cals; 1.2g protein; 5g fat; 2.7g saturated
fat; 16g carbohydrate; 1.1g fibre;
462Kjoules; 12mg cholesterol; 42mg
sodium

p.120 Chocolate Brownies
135cals; 3g protein; 10g fat; 1.5g saturated
fat; 13g carbohydrate; 1.5g fibre;
565Kjoules; 29mg cholesterol; 148mg
sodium

p.121 Easy Irish Soda Bread
142cals; 5.4g protein; 1.9g fat; 0.4g
saturated fat; 27g carbohydrate; 2.9g fibre;
601Kjoules; 0.5mg cholesterol; 219mg
sodium

p.122 Farmhouse Granary Bread
122cals; 5.9g protein; 2.6g fat; 0.3g
saturated fat; 27g carbohydrate; 3.8g fibre;
646Kjoules; 0mg cholesterol; 75mg
sodium

Index

ACKNOWLEDGEMENTS

Index and editorial assistance: Jessica Hughes
Nutritional analysis: Fiona Hunter
Production: Nigel Reed